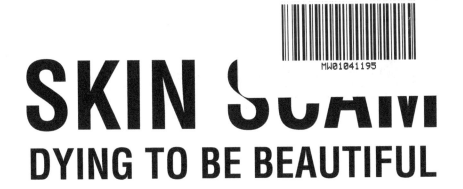

SKIN SCAM
DYING TO BE BEAUTIFUL

MELVIN L. ELSON M.D.

Printed in the United States of America
ISBN: Softcover   978-1-63871-773-7
          Hardback   978-1-63871-774-4
          eBook   978-1-63871-775-1
Republished by: PageTurner Press and Media LLC
Publication Date: 12/03/2021

To order copies of this book, contact:
PageTurner Press and Media
Phone: 1-888-447-9651
info@pageturner.us
www.pageturner.us

SKIN SCAM

Yes, we all know it. The baby boomers are getting older, they don't want to look it, and they are not going to look it. They have never been a generation to sit still and just let things happen. They are also a very powerful force. They made Elvis king. They made Hula-Hoop a favorite toy and had millions eating TV dinners. For that matter, they made TV! Just who are these folks? Baby boomers are that huge group throughout the world born after World War II, between 1946 and the early '60s. Despite the fact that this is a very diverse group, there are certain characteristics shared by all, particularly those in the United States. They like working from home; they take antiaging supplements; and they hate looking old, hate wrinkles, and even hate thinking about getting older. Grow old gracefully—no way! Their hobbies are low-impact sports, particularly those that do not require team participation. They like to be alone and are comfortable with how they live, but not necessarily how they look, and they are going to do something about it. Although they have many thoughts and desires as a group, they are powerful individualists, choosing activities that favor being alone—running, swimming, bicycling, and hiking. You will see youngsters playing football and baseball and octogenarians playing softball, but not baby boomers. No way! Therefore, you see the rise of such industries as Nike, REI, etc.

They tend to overparent, raising trophy children who are the kings and queens, and always get what they want; and the world should pay attention to them because they are worthy as they are the sons and daughters of the baby boomers. On the other hand, they are concerned that they are the last generation in this country that will fare better than their parents did. They are an enigma. They like tailgating, and they like wining and dining, although they do not always have to spend a lot to enjoy them. Their investment of choice is real estate, and their largest investment is their home. They are now beginning to seriously rethink this. They may now stay put rather than move up, and this can be interpreted now as moving up. They still have their home, their biggest investment. They will scrimp and save to splurge on. Private schools are necessary. Get the best for the aging parents, regardless of what it takes; and as far as the family pets are concerned, they are not animals—they are part of the family. Hence, veterinarians now provide hip replacements, cancer chemotherapy, cataract surgery, and on and on for the family dog or cat. Moreover, there is a growth in pet cemeteries. There has been even one family that cloned their beloved dog at a cost of $155,000—anything and everything for the baby boomer and the baby boomer's family. Their emphasis is on tech toys, travel, learning, entertaining, and a proper nest in which to entertain. Creature comforts are necessary at any cost. They will not get older— they must remain in the game. Anything and everything that can be done to keep them looking young and feeling youthful will be done, and they will seek out the ones who can or will do what they want.

In addition, as this generation continues to get older (even though they will not look older), more wealthy and more powerful with their buying power and ability to demand and receive anything and everything they want, those of us in the medical industry (yes, industry) have certainly taken notice. Everyone wants in on the action, whether or not they are qualified and whether or not they even have any training at all. There is now a growing trend of individuals who are not in the medical profession in any way and have never had any type of training participating in the youth craze to keep people looking young—even if they kill them! There is a great deal of money to be made in keeping baby boomers young or at least looking young, and there are some very important issues to look at. Moreover, this is not an issue just for the United States. There is a worldwide explosion of interest; and indeed, demands for cosmetic surgery, cosmetic procedures, products that promise to make us younger or look younger, and all of these are being delivered by a plethora of professionals and nonprofessionals. I have been fortunate enough to teach doctors in fifty different countries how to evaluate and treat the aging face and train them in all types of cosmetic procedures. Many of them are being exposed to the world of aesthetic medicine and surgery for the very first time, even though they may have been in practice in any one of a number of specialties for a number of years. However, not all those who are jumping on the cosmetic baby boomer bandwagon are trained physicians. In addition, these physicians are not all dermatologists and plastic surgeons by any means—they are gynecologists and obstetricians tired of delivering babies and paying outrageous malpractice insurance cost, emergency room doctors who are just tired, and general practitioners who can no longer fight with insurance companies to just get a portion of the fee that they charge and deserve. All kinds of physicians are trying to get into the cosmetic arena that involves very little paperwork, no dealing with insurance, and treating happy patients. However, indeed, many are not physicians at all, and not all patients end up happy. The old adage of selling snake oil has not only returned en masse, but the snake oil that is being sold is sometimes offered by slick snake oil salesmen, the likes of which have never been seen before.

Some of the processes are scientifically valid and proven to be both safe and effective, but not all, and most of the professionals offering these are reputable, honest practitioners of various sorts. We are told we will look younger, feel stronger, have more energy, be more vibrant, be more desirable, finally get the man or woman of our dreams, become wealthy, and on and on and on. What are these hucksters playing on? Our lack of self-esteem. We need to build our self-esteem, self-worth, and value—what we are really all about. A great deal of cosmetic surgery, cosmetic procedures, and cosmetic products is really about increasing self-esteem.

SELF-ESTEEM

How we perceive ourselves and especially how we perceive what others perceive of us may be more important than most of us think it is. It is not only how we look that is important but also how we think we look and how we think other people are thinking about us may be the most important aspect of our lives. One of the most—if not the most important factor in determining how long we will live is actually our self-esteem. Certainly, it plays a big role in how we feel about ourselves and how we interact with others. There is no doubt that appearance plays a key role in our lives because it has been shown in many studies that better-looking people get the best tables in restaurants, get waited on more quickly in department stores, get better jobs, get higher pay, and get faster promotions; but it may surprise you to know that better-looking people get better medical care. And better-looking, more attractive people have a certain swagger. They know they are attractive, and part of what they are able to get in this world may very well be their attitude. I am good-looking, I deserve the best, and I am going to get it! And they do.

A recent article addressed this very well. The article reported that in a recent study, beautiful people are happier, but men and women are so, apparently for different reasons. Handsome men get extra kicks that come from economic benefits, whereas, women are more apt to find joy just looking in the mirror. A study from the University of Texas stated that women just felt that beauty is inherently important, and they just feel bad if they are ugly.

It should also be noted that the pursuit and maintenance of beauty drives a number of huge industries. In 2010, Americans spent $845 million on face-lifts alone. In a recent book, *Beauty Pays*, the author states that a handsome man makes 13 percent more over his career than a looks-challenged man. But interestingly enough, one study showed that those who are unattractive in the workplace may actually have an advantage in that not much is expected of them, and they very well may be able to surpass the low expectations. On the other hand, we have high expectations for the very attractive. We expect Tom Brady to win every football game, and when he loses one, he falls way below our expectations.

Even in nature, in animals, this same phenomenon plays out. An animal born with a slight difference in appearance from other animals in the group is often shunned and allowed to play no role in the running of the society and is not allowed to mate. Now one could argue that this may be a function of control of the good genes so the species does not end up with a perpetuated defect, but there is more to it than just what Darwin would say. An animal that appears to be different may attract attention from predators, as well as cause; however, that does not change how the animal feels! And that has been studied to show that this type of animal—slight defect, e.g., different color than the others—actually becomes depressed, becomes aloof, and eventually has a shorter life span. But what does that have to do with us? As it turns out, a great deal.

At the moment, this country is full of sad, depressed, overworked, sleep-deprived, obese people; and this affects absolutely everything that we do. If one can control perhaps one aspect—say, a line on the forehead—then not only is that improvement in appearance, but it is something more. It is in a way a method of saying, "I can control something." Not the terrorists, not the gas prices, not the economy, etc.

Another aspect that is extremely important to our longevity and our quality of life is our nutritional status—or lack thereof. The National Institute of Health and the US Department of Agriculture conducted surveys to determine what percentage of Americans actually ate a healthy diet to the point of stating that the diet was healthy, was nutritious, and met all the requirements set up as standards for American diet. The answer? Not one person of the over sixteen thousand people surveyed over a two-year period. Some did have adequate levels of some vitamins (most commonly B12), and most had very low levels of some other nutrients such as zinc. Even more frightening was the fact that only 20 percent women had an adequate amount of folate—a very important nutrient to prevent birth defects. This—coupled with our lack of exercise, obesity, fast-food fetish, smoking, etc.—leads to a population that is aging faster than we should and can easily reverse the process. There are many things we can do to look better, feel better, and live longer; and it really does not take that much effort. Stop smoking. Get off the couch, and take steps toward proper nutrition with not only good eating habits but also proper supplementation. Stop killing yourself!

Although not yet well known, there have been great strides made in the areas of nutrition as well as methods of accurately measuring our nutritional status. One of the most important concepts that has come out of a great deal of research in many different university settings is the fact that a great deal of aging comes about because of something called free radicals. To begin understanding the real basis for nutrition and why and how we age, it is necessary to delve into a little bit of science.

Obviously, we cannot live without oxygen, but it is this very basic part of life that contributes a great deal to our aging and forms the basis of an understanding of nutritional status. When we utilize oxygen as a fuel, the leftover part of the molecule forms what is known as a free radical, and this free radical is like a snowball that has been pushed off the top of a hill. It just keeps rolling and knocking down everything in its path. In scientific terms, it has set up a cascade that leads to cell damage. As this occurs repeatedly and is based on our use of oxygen, there are substances that can be utilized to reverse and fight this process—the so-called antioxidants. Some of these are more familiar to you than others such as vitamins C, E, and A. These really form the first line of defense against free radicals, but there are many others such as lutein (found in tomatoes), lycopene (same), alpha lipoic acid, and many others. The more antioxidants we have, the better able we are to fight off the ravages of the free radicals. These are not only derived from the use of oxygen but also increased by smoking and pollution.

But then again, what about the way we look? That is a huge part of our self-esteem and is dependent on all the factors already mentioned, and you had better believe there are so many people waiting to sell you so many things and do so much to you. So who are these characters?

I will cover nutrition, exercise, weight control, and other methods that make you live longer, healthier, fuller, prettier lives; but what about the outside?

Moreover, what are we trying to achieve anyway? What is youth? What is beauty? Keats said, "Beauty is truth, truth beauty—that is all ye know on earth, and all ye need to know." The concept of beauty has evolved over the centuries. When one looks at Venus of Willendorf, which is actually a fertility figure, it is certainly not our vision of beauty. In addition, there are differences across cultural lines. There are still tribes in Africa that consider huge stretched lips a thing of beauty— much more so than in *First Wives Club*—and there are also those who stretch the neck over time to allow many rings to be placed. However, in the modern era, there are generally a few items that contribute to what is considered a beautiful face that transcends all cultures.

A woman should have an oval face, arched eyebrows, a clear skin, and a good demarcation between the face and the neck; and in actuality, when you see a beautiful woman, all you see are the eyes and the lips. Think of any beautiful woman. What does her nose look like? You do not remember, and it does not matter. The reason a person has a nose job performed is that the nose is in the way. It should not be seen, and in the perfect face, it really is not. A face-lift is performed because the picture has slipped out of the frame, and it needs to be put back—anything that detracts from the eyes and the lips has to go. Same reasoning goes for getting rid of dark spots and blemishes on the face; it detracts from what we really want to see.

When viewing an attractive man, the emphasis is not the same. The face is quite different with it being squarer, lower forehead, no arch to the eyebrows, and almost no lips. The most important thing is the gaze, the way he looks at you. Think of George Clooney or James Bond, you are being engaged by the man, and that attracts you to him.

These are some of the characteristics that apply to making the baby boomer woman and man appear attractive and perhaps young. How do we do that?

Life was so simple in the good old days, only ten to fifteen years ago. You took care of your skin by going to the cosmetic counter. The young woman in the white coat would sell you a moisturizer, and your skin actually felt better and maybe even looked a little better. You could go to a spa and receive a facial and some pampering that made you feel better all over, more beautiful, and more youthful. This could be repeated as often as you wanted, and there were even products you could buy there to keep you gorgeous! Moreover, the bottles were so beautiful, and the packaging was so pretty. And the products are actually just moisturizers. Nevertheless, such great moisturizers! At $50–200 a jar, they should be. There is now a department store moisturizer that sells for $799.

A new era began in the late 1980s, when physicians came into the beauty market. How did this occur? Well, very simple. Dermatologists were already well aware of the fact that most of what is called aging by the general public is really sun damage, and while in the process of preventing skin cancer with the use of sunscreens as well as new products that came to the fore, the visible signs of aging were also decreased. Then the miracle in the tube arrived upon the scene.

Back in the 1960s and before, dermatologists treated many disorders, including complexion problems and acne, with high doses of vitamin

A. It did not take too long to figure out that the skin was clearing up and doing nicely, but since vitamin A is a fat-soluble vitamin, the liver was not able to handle all the vitamin A it was expected to store. Thus began the search for a way to apply vitamin A to the skin so that the benefit could be obtained without the horrendous side effects. But alas, vitamin A was too unstable to put into a formula that could be used on the skin. The difficult search then began, looking for a way to try to use this compound and have it both stable and effective for a period when used on the skin. Dr. Albert Kligman of the University of Pennsylvania came up with the answer. Instead of using vitamin A, which is an alcohol, he developed a form of vitamin A acid also known as Retin-A* that was stable in the formula and was effective on the skin to treat acne.

Retin-A was approved in the late '60s by the FDA for the treatment of acne and, although somewhat irritating, became the standard treatment for acne around the world. Over the next few decades, many physicians, including Dr. Kligman, began to notice, and patients began to report, that their lines, wrinkles, mottled discoloration, and sallowness of the skin began to improve. This led to the announcement on *NBC Nightly News* in the mid-1980s that Retin-A was the new miracle cream for the treatment of aging skin, and the new era of cosmeceuticals was born—substances used on the skin from both the cosmetic and pharmaceutical industry that were shown to benefit aging skin. It is important to realize that this term, as far as the FDA is concerned, does not exist; but it does and refers to products that are from the cosmetic arena that definitely have an effect on the skin, particularly in improving the appearance of aging and wrinkles. These are not products that are approved by the FDA. FDA approves only drugs, yet they are more than cosmetics because they do much more than just adorn the skin—they treat and interact with it.

Before going any further, this is a good jump-off point to begin to find out what really causes aging of the skin. I think it is important for anyone who is considering improving your appearance and embarking on the road of life-long self-improvement to understand what can and cannot be done and the role played in treating the various aspects of aging, particularly the aging face. You cannot delay a face-lift by applying creams to the skin, and you cannot get smooth, wrinkle-free, perfect skin with a face-lift!

Figure 1 is a patient I saw more than twenty years ago, whose face demonstrates all the factors of the aging face.

The aging face is made up of five factors, and it does not make any difference if you are eighteen or eighty. There are only five factors that can influence the aging face. The first factor is intrinsic aging. That means the skin simply wears out. Like everything else, it simply gets old. The interesting thing is that skin doesn't even begin to truly wear out until around age seventy and if you see someone who is really old, say ninety or one hundred, it is obvious. What the face looks like is that there is a thin piece of parchment overhanging a skull that is shrinking because that is really what is happening. The skin loses much of the underlying fat support, and the lower skin (the dermis) actually thins out. However, amazingly, the skull actually does get smaller over time.

You can see from the picture that there is some thinning of the skin just under the eyes, over the cheekbones. This is the only manifestation in this sixty-year-old patient of intrinsic aging.

Although there is not a great deal of desire to treat this particular aspect of the aging face because of the chronological age usually involved, there is treatment available. Implants of many different types can be either surgically placed under the skin or injected, and fat movement or transplant from another area of the body can provide a pleasing full appearance. Additionally, with the newer filling materials that have become available, the face can be contoured and made to look younger and smoother (like reflating a deflated balloon). Some type of surgical intervention could be of significant benefit in treating this aspect of the aging face. It should also be noted that intrinsic aging will occur in younger individuals who smoke due to decreased circulation in the small blood vessels of the skin, so again, to avoid true aging, avoid smoking.

The second factor is one that is rarely considered by the patient or the physician in discussing the changing face, and that is sleep lines. Sleep lines etch the surface of the skin in the same manner that a napkin gets a fold when kept in the same position in a drawer over time. All of us find a position in which to sleep that is most comfortable for us, and that position remains the same—night after night, week after week, year in and year out. This is also true with the position of the face on, in, or even around a pillow. The same stress on the skin tends to produce a fold or line because of the stress on the same area again and again, just like the napkin. These lines are really quite interesting, strange, but interesting. They look like they do not make sense. They occur on one side of the face. Men tend to get them on the forehead, and they appear diagonally across the lines going across the forehead from one side to the other. Women, on the other hand, get them on the cheeks and along the chin, moving diagonally across other lines. These lines are bothersome and can get deeper and deeper over time. In this patient, the sleep line is located on the left side of the chin, moving diagonally across the area crossing many other lines.

There are pillows that are made to hold the head in one position to decrease sleep lines. I am not sure if the decrease caused by keeping the face out of the same sleeping position, or it just will not let you sleep. Satin pillowcases are also available, and these are beneficial as well, since the skin tends to slide over the case and not stick in the same position. I have not found it possible to have patients change their sleeping pattern to rid themselves of these lines because once you are asleep, you revert to the pattern that is most comfortable and familiar to you. Some significant numbers of women sleep with a pillow on their chest, and this causes vertical lines to occur between the breasts, which is easily treated with Botox.

The third factor is gravity. Once we stand up, everything moves toward the ground! The upper eyelids come over the eyes, the lower lids puff out and thin, allowing the dark circles to form, the jowls form, the tip of the nose points more toward the ground and so does the chin. The upper lip seems to disappear. Where has it gone? It is inside the mouth! Take a look in the mirror and get out a picture of your wedding or prom or sometime when you were years younger, and notice how much smaller and thinner your upper lip is. The lower lip pouts out more, and as the chin continues in its downward spiral, a line begins to form that was never there before—the chin crease. In addition, the neck produces the turkey waddle, and even the ears get longer.

Notice in this figure, the upper eyelids have moved down, the lower lids have also moved downward, allowing the dark circle and thin skin to form under the eyelids. Additionally, the tip of the nose is pointing to the ground rather than straight ahead. The upper lip is small, the lower lip has moved down and out, creating the pout and line of the chin, and the chin has become very prominent.

If you want to see how much gravity has affected your skin, lie on the bed with your head off the side and look in the mirror. You will be amazed. So what in the world can be done about this look? In actuality, quite a bit, although this is the most difficult of all the factors in the aging face to address. Any factor due to significant gravity changes can be treated by surgical means. However, there is a great change that is occurring now in how the aging face is assessed and therefore what methods are used to treat it. Still, with the exception of contouring the face with filling materials, almost every method is surgical. The most common surgical procedure performed over the last few decades and even until today is the face-lift. There is a reason for this. If you can consider the face as a canvas on which all the factors paint their part of the picture, gravity makes the face slip off the canvas. The picture is no longer framed and must be fixed. Up until recently, the only procedure used was the classical face-lift, where the excess skin is cut off and what remains is pulled into place to give a lifting appearance, placing the picture back into the frame. Sounds familiar? If you have ever baked a pie, the excess crust is trimmed off and then the crust fits the pie! Now a concept has finally taken hold that should have been obvious long ago, and that is the fact that a child's face is not pulled tight. All of us know people who have had multiple face-lifts and begin to look like a bird instead of a human. People are not pointed. They are round, and the younger we are, the more round and full are the youthful face. That has given birth to procedures that do more than just pull the skin and redrape it. As the skin is fitted back into place, the underlying fat should be moved to its original location also. So fat is moved around under the skin to make a round full appearance, like a baby's face! Even more recently, procedures have been developed that allow some of the newer injectable materials to be placed into the skin in such a manner that it lifts the skin back into place and rounds out the face, creating a more youthful appearance. Some marketing has been done that refers to this procedure as a liquid face-lift.

There are many surgical procedures available to treat the gravity factor of the face. From a nose job to round out the falling pointed tip, to chin enhancement, and certainly many procedures available to change the aging lips back to their youthful appearance. As we age, the shifting that occurs with gravity makes the upper lip become smaller than the lower lip as it shifts inside the mouth. A more youthful look can be obtained with many of the myriad of injectable materials available around the world, and we will discuss many of these later; but for now, just look at your lips and go find that picture of you when you went to the prom or your wedding photo and compare the two. That can be changed!

There are so many things that can be done these days; there is even a procedure that decreases the length of the ears that have gotten longer over time.

The fourth factor in changing the face over time consists of expression lines, lines that occur from muscles pulling on the same collagen fibers repeatedly to produce the lines particularly around the eyes and the mouth, extending from the nose to the lips and on the forehead. Until the last few years, the only reasonable treatment was to inject these with some type of filling material, but the miracle of Botox has appeared. However, there are nuances to all this. Botox or any of the newer botulinum toxins for injections is not the answer for all lines and wrinkles by any means and needs to be really understood as to how, why, and where this can and cannot be used. We will discuss both the available fillers around the world and Botox in a separate chapter. At this point, it is enough to say that there is a very good, effective, and safe treatment for lines occurring over the face if done properly by the right people.

The last factor in the aging face is really the one that most of us refer to when we evaluate someone's appearance as old, and that is the sun. In actuality, at least 70 percent of what is classified as aging is sun damage, and that doesn't even take into consideration the other problem associated with the effects of sun on the skin—cancer. However, getting back to aging skin. To see the effects of the sun on your skin is really very easy. Just look at the back of your hands and compare them with the top of your feet. On the other hand, compare the appearance of the youthful skin of the buttock cheek with the aged skin of the cheeks on the face. They are the same age, but they do not look alike. The skin that has not been exposed to the sun has remained smooth, wrinkle free, and uniform in color, like a baby's butt. However, the sun exposed skin produces so many things—lines, wrinkles, coarseness, so many different colors and textures! There is a reason that the process of turning the skin of a cow into leather is called *tanning*. All of the effects of the sun on the skin are bad. Look at what it does to the furniture that is in the sun or your drapes or your car. The list goes on and on, yet you can still walk down on any beach in the world and see people of all ages with as much skin as can be exposed to get that healthy golden glow. Well, it is not at all healthy, and we really have no reason to get out in the sun. It is unfortunate that since this accounts for the majority of what is referred to as aging and is easily manipulated, it is the factor that attracts skin care products, most of which do nothing but moisturize and promise things that cannot come true. There are a few things that actually do have an effect, and we will discuss it in detail. Therefore, these are the factors of the aging face, simply how and why we age. Moreover, everyone wants a piece of the action. There are so many ways to make money in treating aging and the appearance of aging. There are the cosmetic companies, the drug companies, the aestheticians, and all types of doctors who are trying to treat aging and all kinds of ways to get information. Sure, there are consultations available from doctors. Are they the most reliable source? Maybe, maybe not. And of course, there is that bastion of all knowledge—the Internet. And for those who can't sleep and have nothing better to do, you can certainly buy products from the myriad of infomercials plying their wares that guarantee you to look better, live longer, be stronger, sexier, and richer. You name it, and they will allow you to give them your credit card number to send you all kinds of wonderful things. I am going to let you in on a few things, some of the real secrets. I have practiced medicine and cosmetic dermatology for over twenty-five years, have consulted with drug and cosmetic companies the world over, developed skin care lines, performed all types of research, started cosmetic companies, and even done infomercials. Most of the information out there is false or at least significantly exaggerated. A significant number of the guarantees are frauds, and many of the doctors have no training or expertise that you think they do. (Some of them are not even doctors!)

As we move forward in this exercise, we will go into detail as to who should and who should not be touching your skin. What procedures and products work, and which are just marketing swindles. There is the who, what, where, how, and when. So let us get started with the who.

WHO SHOULD TOUCH YOU?

What do you do if your car will not run properly? Obviously, if you are going to drive, you need to get it fixed. In addition, it does not matter a great deal whether you own an old beat-up hunk of a car or a new Bentley; you are going to go to an expert of some sort to get the work done. You are not going to go to any car repair shop to get the repairs done. So what about your body, especially your face? Certainly, there are many people who want to do all types of things to you, and it is difficult to discern what is real and what is not.

Plastic surgeons are generally held in great regard when it comes to evaluating and treating the aging face, and how well they should be. They have been at the forefront of what to do and how to do it when it comes to the aging face for decades. However, things are changing. Plastic surgeons—some called aesthetic or cosmetic surgeons, but those who are real plastic surgeons, i.e., certified by the American Board of Plastic Surgeons—are trained to spend their time and effort and skills in the operating room. They have learned that not every patient wants or needs to be cut, so they have added other services—selling all types of skin care products that they, and probably the staff, know very little, if anything, about. They are trained by a salesperson to sell as much as they can to whomever, and the office knows if they can get someone in there to start buying products, then they can also start doing minor procedures such as injections and peels and then laser, and finally, they are where they were intended to be herded all the time—in the operating room, getting the procedure. Remember, a surgeon cuts, and he cuts under the skin. It is like a room with a door. The surgeon is in the room, but that does not make him an expert on the door! The great majority of plastic surgeons really know very little about skin care, aging skin, or anything about how to actually treat the skin. That is not what they have been trained to do. They are surgeons, and surgeons cut. You cannot rely on them for advice on anything to do with skin care. They may or may not have knowledgeable ancillary personnel working for them, performing minor procedures and selling skin care products. But what is the point? You go to a plastic surgeon for surgery, and there are other doctors who are really the experts in treating aging skin and that, of course, are the dermatologist.

However, plastic surgeons are not the only ones who have smelled opportunity here. Of course, there are the dermatologists, who are the experts on the skin. Unfortunately, until recently, they were really the experts on skin disease, from diaper rash to skin cancer to nail fungus. Only over the last decade or so has the dermatologist stepped to the forefront and started caring for healthy skin to keep it healthy as well as treating aging skin as disease and reversing the process using all types of remedies at his disposal—certainly lotions and potions, but also chemical peels, injections of filling agents, laser resurfacing, and the ubiquitous Botox. Some dermatologists have gone even further and are performing eye jobs, liposuction, and even face-lifts. Now it is true that some dermatologists are very skilled in these more invasive procedures, and some have operating rooms in the office that are approved and have everything necessary to keep the patient comfortable and safe. *But* that is not what the dermatologists spent in all those years of training. In my opinion, face-lifts, tummy tucks, neck lifts, etc., should be done by the most qualified who have the greatest likelihood of being well trained; and that is the plastic surgeon. Surgical training with a background in general surgery is where the plastic surgeon learns how to deal not only with things when all goes well, but when things don't go well. Dermatologists do not have this type of training in their background.

Dermatologists are trained for many years to treat problems of the skin, and this now includes all the aspects of skin aging. Injection of filling materials is no different from any of the other myriads of items dermatologists have been injecting into the skin for centuries. Dermabrasion, chemical peels, and laser resurfacing are merely different *methods of wounding the skin in various ways and allowing it to heal smoother and prettier and appear more youthful.* All these things are in the area of dermatology. Certainly, there are procedures learned from other specialties such as injection of Botox, which was devised by ophthalmologists in conjunction with dermatologist (actually, the first to do this procedure was a husband-and-wife team of an ophthalmologist and a dermatologist, Drs. Jean and Alastair Carruthers of Vancouver, British Columbia, Canada).

This brings us to another point, and that is not only who should be doing procedures on you, but where should they be done. True, common sense tells most people not to line up outside the door of a hotel room in Miami to let someone from out of the country inject an unknown substance to increase the size of their lips or inject their wrinkles, but they do. Common sense should tell most people not to get together in a bar or a restaurant with a group so they can get Botox injected, but they do. I even saw a sign for a Botox party in a sushi bar in Berlin! Now there is a combination. But getting back to the operating room, there are, of course, many operating rooms in hospitals; but now there are also freestanding surgery centers, and many doctors have operating rooms in their offices. Some have the operating room in the office for convenience of the doctor and patient as well as cutting down on the cost for the patient while at the same time increasing the profit for the physician's office. There is absolutely nothing wrong with this as long as the operating room is approved and certified, just as the doctor should be board certified, which is a stamp of approval by his peers that he has the qualifications to perform procedures, treat diseases, etc. for which he has been trained. In other words, he knows what he is doing. The same is true for the operating room. It should be certified that it meets all the requirements of the agencies such as Medicare and state agencies, that it is fully equipped and maintained for your safety and comfort in the event that everything goes well, and even more important, in the event that it doesn't.

You may think it is a simple thing for anyone to get operating room privileges in the hospital, and you may think it is simple to set up an operating room in the office and get it approved for use. In actuality, all of these things are very difficult. Hospitals and the surgeons who operate in them are very protective of the operating rooms and with who is allowed to be associated with them, and in my opinion, that is the way it should be. True, it has led to some serious turf battles, keeping doctors who may have had some training by fellowship and are qualified to perform some procedures out of the operating room, but it does tend to keep out those doctors who have not undergone the rigorous training of the surgical specialist. This is part of the reason that operating rooms are becoming more and more common in various doctors' offices. But you have to be careful. Setting up an operating room and getting it approved is not the same thing. If you are considering undergoing any procedure in an outpatient setting, particularly an office of a physician, you need to be certain that that facility is approved by a government agency—Medicare and/or state offices. The doctor does not have to be a Medicare provider to have the operating room approved by Medicare. That is one of the jobs of this particular government agency. That is no guarantee that everything will go well, but it is certainly a step in the right direction. On the other hand, if approvals are not in place, you do not need to ask why;

you just need to seek help elsewhere. Just like the board certification that I briefly mentioned. When a physician completes residency and/or fellowship in a specialty, that doctor becomes board eligible. That means he is now able to take an examination—usually written and oral and very difficult—to prove his proficiency in the specialty. Many specialties today repeat examinations for doctors every five years so that doctors can demonstrate that they are still up to date on the latest advances in that particular specialty. If a doctor takes the board exam and fails it, he is still board eligible for a period but not board certified. It is important for you to choose a doctor who is board certified, just as you would choose a certified mechanic to work on your car.

So we have the dermatologist as the expert in the skin and now beginning to come to the fore as the expert in treating a new disease—skin aging, and that is entirely appropriate. In addition, we have the plastic surgeon who has been trained with a surgical background and can help you with invasive procedures such as a face-lift. Great! But where are all these other doctors coming from? Why are gynecologists performing cosmetic procedures? Because they know women? I don't think so. Certainly, you trust your family doctor, your pediatrician, your gynecologist, but that does not give them or you the right or the obligation to let them perform procedures that they learned from a seminar or a representative of the company selling a product or procedure or getting training from the manual that comes with a machine such as a laser. Use your head! Use common sense! You would not want your dermatologist to fill your teeth. Why would you let your dentist inject something for wrinkles? You don't want me delivering your baby. Why should your ob-gyn inject Botox? Because he knows you? I don't think so.

This arena of many different medical specialists performing treatments for aging skin is one that is very complicated and becoming more and more of an issue around the world. Certainly, there are situations in which you cannot have access to a dermatologist or plastic surgeon and need the services of one of the so-called noncore physicians. It is then that you need a great deal of more information about what you are getting into, but you cannot always choose the best-case scenario of having a plastic surgeon performing your face-lift, a facial plastic surgeon doing your nose job, a dermatologist injecting filling materials and laser therapy, and the aesthetician pampering you with facials. It just isn't that simple anymore.

Then after the doctors, you have an entire array of individuals who are there to help you with your cosmetic desires. There are aestheticians, nurses, nurse practitioners, and physician assistants. Sure, there are also people out there who have no qualifications at all; but for now, let's look at people who are qualified to do some things and where they may be located and trained that meets your needs and safety requirements.

First, the aesthetician. This is interesting because it is a diverse group of people, many of whom are very qualified, well-trained, and knowledgeable, but there are also those that somehow fit into this category but really don't belong there. I once asked the State of Tennessee for a list of all the aestheticians licensed in the state, and I received a list of thousands of people, some of whom worked in spas and performed procedures such as facials and chemical peels and who were doing hair out of their houses. When I asked about the disparity, I was told that this was a list of anyone not licensed as a nurse or physician who is allowed to touch someone in the state of Tennessee. And there are many other states that have the same ruling in place. On the other hand, there are states, such as New Jersey, that are very strict and do an excellent job policing those who are allowed access to the human body.

For the most part, aestheticians are trained to perform some very minor procedures on the skin, from facials to enzyme peels and even some chemical peels. I know that a number of years ago, I worked with a company to develop a skin-care line with a chemical peel for both aestheticians and physicians. The chemical peel that was developed for the aesthetician market was much milder than the one for the physicians. Our primary goal was to make certain that the procedure could not hurt anyone. Not that it had to be effective, just not harmful. So what was the purpose of even having one to sell products? The peel was a means to get the client involved and then buy products to keep the benefits going. This is not unusual at all in this segment of the cosmetic industry, and it is something to keep in mind as you are evaluating what you really want and what you really need. As far as this goes for the aesthetician, there is no problem with what they are doing with facials, selling products, and performing these mild procedures such as the enzyme and mild chemical peels. One of the significant problems occurs when they overstep their boundaries. Some aestheticians are in effect practicing medicine by performing medium-depth peels, laser treatments, and even injecting collagen and other fillers and even Botox for wrinkles. There is nowhere in this country that this practice is legal, but it is done. Be careful! Know who is treating you! You cannot believe the marketing that is out there in this area. I have seen advertisements stating that an aesthetician is certified by the FDA in doing laser procedures. The FDA does not certify anyone to do anything; that is not the job of the agency. The FDA approves drugs, devices, and biological materials and follows them to be certain that they remain safe after entering the market. The FDA has nothing to do with determining the qualifications of any individual—aesthetician, doctor, nurse, or anyone else.

So who are all these people, crowding into the medical field of treatment of the aging face?

Physician assistants come from many areas of discipline, and it doesn't have to even be related to medicine and take special training and work under the control of a physician and a guidebook. Some are very proficient at what they do and become very well trained and very experienced. As a matter of fact, one of the best injectors of materials for wrinkles and Botox that I know is a physician's assistant in Detroit. You may actually be getting treatments now from a physician's assistant under the direction of a physician and not even know it. But that is OK. There should be no problem as long as the caregiver is trained, and the physician is on the premises, and *you* know what is going on. You are informed!

Then there are the nurses—LPNs, RNs, and nurse practitioners. LPN stands for licensed practical nurse. These individuals usually take a couple of years training and work with patients to provide basic care such as bathing, taking blood pressure and temperature, and giving meds, but some have become highly skilled through years of experience in a particular field, and I have seen situations in which they are providing care such as injecting collagen, assisting with laser procedures, and many other things. RNs have been the backbone of medical care for hundreds of years, but unfortunately, many nursing schools closed over the last decade or so due to lack of funds, and this important link in medical care has become less and less common. In addition, due to the immense problems with paperwork from the government and the insurance companies, many of these highly skilled and well-trained individuals are pushing paper. However, I digress. These nurses in doctors' offices are performing many procedures, from laser to vein injections to soft tissue augmentation to Botox and on and on and on, and they are, in my opinion, quite qualified to work in the office but not necessarily directly under the doctor's supervision at all times.

The nurse practitioner is supposed to be another step past the RN in training, licensing, and the ability to work independently. The initial idea was that these professionals would work in rural areas, delivering babies, providing prenatal care, etc. This position, which is very important in the delivery of medical care, has evolved over the years. There are many nurse practitioners in physicians' offices delivering excellent health care in the cosmetic surgery arena—assisting in surgery, performing soft tissue augmentation with all types of filling agents, injecting Botox, treating leg veins, some having their own practices specializing in one area or another within the office. However, I recently learned that there are no requirements in the area of nursing for someone to take the graduate courses and become a nurse practitioner. This was brought out very succinctly when I saw a nurse practitioner drop an instrument on the floor during surgery and just pick it up to be used. I asked her about her experience in the hospital, etc. as a nurse and found out that she had no nursing background at all. She was clueless as to what to do in the operating room, how to handle medicines or anything else. She expected to be trained on the job. This is not only ludicrous, it is dangerous! She was actually surprised when I would not train her to inject Restylane* and Botox* even thought she had no clue as to how to even mix the Botox to get it ready for injection.

These individuals, from the licensed aesthetician to the nurse practitioner, can be very helpful when they stick to what they are supposed to do and have proper training; and just like physicians, they vary in their ability to provide care. However, another group needs to be addressed before we go on, and that is the individual who has no training to do anything, no qualifications, no license, and no intention of ever helping anyone. Their only aim is to make money and to make it quickly. These are people who come into the United States from various locations (or are from here), mostly south of the border, set up a shop in a hotel room, usually in Los Angeles or Miami, stay for a day, and perform some type of cosmetic procedure, usually injecting something for wrinkles. It used to be thought that these people were injecting silicone, but it is now known that they are injecting all types of substances into the unsuspecting faces, even blood or dirt. They will do anything and inject all types of things to make money, and then they are gone. They advertise in the local paper that they are going to be there, or they use word of mouth (safer for them), to do their business, and then they are gone. In addition, the demand is so great that you can barely get in the door for all the people waiting in line! How utterly stupid! As of this writing, Miami-Dade police have established a special task force to look into this very problem. It has become so prevalent that an entire part of this police force goes after these perpetrators, and they are finding them every day.

But what about the qualified, well-trained doctor who is supposed to be looking out after the interests of the patient before anything else? What about him? Well, there are still many of them around, but there are also those who have seen the opportunity of the aging baby boomer and her pocketbook to fill his wallet. And they are in all specialties. Although I have mentioned those licensed physicians who are expanding beyond the specialty for which they trained, such as gynecologists performing cosmetic surgery (on the face), what about the doctors who are trained in their specialty and wanted to keep others out of their so-called territory? I own this patient, and you had better stay away! Is any of that going on too? You had better believe it—the turf battle.

THE TURF BATTLE

This is a huge problem in the cosmetic surgery and cosmetic medical specialties. Although there are a number of specialties represented here, the battle is raging between only two groups—the dermatologist and the plastic surgeon. And it does not only have the individual doctors involved, but also the societies that represent them. They have even hired marketing firms and PR firms to make sure that what belongs to them, *you*, are kept out of the hands of the others. Why?

Probably there are some who strongly believe in what they are doing and know that what they are doing to protect themselves and their patients is right, but it is mostly about money. In addition, I am sure that is no surprise to you. The battle is fought around two facts: Plastic surgeons spend most of their time in the operating room, in either the hospital or the office, but still they are cutting. That is what they are trained to do, and that is what they do best. One way to make more money is to have someone in the office doing minor noninvasive procedures such as collagen injections (the so-called nurse injector) and selling skin care products.

OK, so what is the other side of the problem? Dermatologists are skin doctors. Originally, the specialty evolved to treat people with skin disease, from diaper rash to psoriasis to skin cancer; but over the last couple of decades, the specialty has turned more and more to the cosmetic aspect of the specialty, treating aged and aging skin. A disease? Maybe. At any rate, most dermatologists do not undergo rigorous surgical training and few are allowed on the staff of hospitals to perform surgery. Nevertheless, some dermatologists are performing surgery, and some have a great deal of training by working with specialists in the field and taking fellowships and the like. However, here comes the problem. They are not allowed to perform surgery in the hospital, so they set up surgical suites in the office. However, these must have the approval of the various state and federal agencies to be up and running. Therefore, here is the scenario: Plastic surgeons want nurses and other personnel to do procedures in the office that dermatologists often do, and dermatologists want to do some of the surgical procedures that plastic surgeons do. *Not on my watch.* So what do they do? Plastic surgeons have launched campaigns, some of them vicious in various state houses, etc. to make it a law that if a doctor is not allowed to perform surgery in a hospital, he should not be allowed to perform that procedure in his office, and if he is attempting to set up an operating room in his office, it should not be allowed.

Conversely, the American Academy for Dermatologic Surgery launched a campaign to disparage procedures performed by anyone but physicians. A survey was sent out to all members (of which I was one) and asked to list the side effects and all the problems seen by the physicians caused by treatment by nonphysicians. I thought this was grossly unfair. When I discussed with the marketing team at the ASDS that most of the problems I see are from other physicians I was told they were not interested in that, only problems by paramedical personnel. Shortly thereafter, I resigned from that society. Therefore, you have a situation in which dermatologists object to any personnel except doctors and plastic surgeons performing procedures of any type, wanting only trained surgeons who are admitted to hospitals to operate on the premises and be able to perform surgical procedures. Both sides state that all of these concerns are for the benefit of the patient, but I think anyone can see through that without any difficulty at all.

What can you do with all these things going on? Be careful, ask questions, and demand to know what the qualifications are, how many procedures have been done by that person, and look at the before and after pictures of their results. They may not tell the truth, but you can at least ask; and if you are not totally comfortable with the answers that you are getting, go somewhere else. As a matter of fact, it is never a bad idea to seek at least two opinions on anything you are considering having done or even on products you are thinking of using on your skin.

However, there can be a bad apple in any bunch. There seems to be a plethora of young doctors now who are coming out of training wanting nothing but to make money. I know that many people think that is what most doctors are interested in, but that is not really the case at all. Most doctors really put the welfare of their patients first and know that they are not going to starve. The income will be there. So what if the doctor is only after money? Can't he still help you? Maybe, but maybe not. In addition, how can you really tell if he is interested in you and not your money and that he can help you? There are a number of things that will tip you off. You certainly cannot tell anything about a doctor's credentials by simply looking in the yellow pages. As a matter of fact, that is the worst place to look. So you were referred by your personal doctor to the specialist to help with your appearance, and that should be on the up and up. Most likely, yes, but sometimes doctors simply refer to their golfing or country club friends and do not know a lot about them. The best place to get a referral to a doctor you want to see regarding your appearance is from family and friends who have seen this doctor. Once you are in, there are still some items that should not be overlooked before you come under his or her care. What if it took you a long time to get an appointment? That is a good sign, isn't it? After all, good restaurants are booked up well in advance. What about doctors? Well, he may have been out of town for a few days or weeks; he may only see certain types of patients on certain days. In addition, you do not know whether he tries to see ten or one hundred patients a day and whether or not he spends time with you or his staff. They may even do most of the procedures. So what do you do? *Ask questions.* He is not a god on a pedestal, and you deserve to know as much about him as possible before you consent to anything. Ask how many of these types of procedures has he done and where he trained. What types of side effects or problems has he had? If he says he has not had any, then that is a real red flag. Every doctor and every procedure does involve the possibility of side effects, and as a good friend of mine who is an expert in treating the aging face says, "If you sand enough wood, you are going to get some splinters." No doctor can share the names of patients with you to talk with, but they can show you before and after pictures of the work they do and not the results in textbooks or brochures. If the doctor tells you that he will get your insurance to pay for a cosmetic procedure, this is another red flag, and you should run—not walk—to the nearest exit. He is dishonest and will not treat you *honestly and fairly.* Most likely, he will not treat you well. I am very familiar with one doctor who does this very thing. He tells patients that he will get the insurance company to pay for the cosmetic procedure by falsifying the documentation. The patient thinks that is so fortunate and so nice of the doctor. If he, however, is dishonest in this area, you can bet he has problems in other areas. Unfortunately, you do not know you are in trouble until you have a side effect or problem and then try to get him to straighten things out. He blames you or simply will not address the matter and says that whatever it is, it will go away eventually. This is the time to switch doctors even though it may be too late. If he spends seconds with you and then turns you over to his well-trained assistant, this is another indication that you have chosen the wrong doctor. Basically, what is important is to find a doctor who can demonstrate that he is well trained in the procedure for which you are looking, will share results with you, discuss openly and honestly both the results and the possible side effects as well as the true cost and how it is to be paid. You also need to know if he, not his office, is going to do the procedure, be in charge of ancillary issues such as skin care, and that you can talk to him and relate to him. You must choose not only a good doctor, but also a good physician.

OK. We have looked at who is doing things to you and how to go about working through that as best as you can. What about the things they are doing and the products you are buying from doctors, specialty stores, spas, catalogues, and even infomercials? Let us look at what works, what doesn't work, and what might even be dangerous!

There are three categories into which topical preparations fit. Drugs are those substances that when applied to the skin, interact with the normal mechanism of the skin or its response and change the way the skin behaves. For example, hydrocortisone is a drug, and whether it is obtained in lower dosages without a prescription or in higher concentrations that require a prescription, there is no question that it is a drug. Cosmetics, on the other hand, adorn the skin, do not interact with it, and have no influence on the way it behaves. Powder is a good example. In addition, this simple dichotomy was the way it was and the Cosmetics and Toiletries Act of 1933 established it, but things were destined not to remain so simple. It became more complicated with the introduction of a new term by Dr. Albert Kligman (inventor of Retin-A)—cosmeceuticals. Dermatologists and others use this category in the cosmetic industry to define those substances that are not drugs that are effective in changing the skin. This is obviously a gray area, and FDA does not recognize the term. It does not mean it does not exist; it just means it is not recognized.

In addition, as we look at all the creams and lotions and potions you can use and the procedures that you can undergo, only scientific evidence will be used to determine whether you are being treated or tricked. Marketing data is no good. Claims that are not substantiated by scientific study are no good. Anecdotal data, for example, claims based on experience in the marketplace from a great number of users may or may not be valid. We will just have to analyze these one by one. So let us look.

VITAMIN A—THE SKIN VITAMIN

*V*itamin A (retinol) was discovered in 1913. It was initially found in milk and cheese, but is contained in many types of meats and green leafy vegetables as well as carrots and other orange, yellow, and red vegetables. It is necessary for vision as well as proper function of skin and bone. It has a rather interesting saga in the treatment of the skin. Back in the 1950s and '60s dermatologists treated a wide variety of ailments with vitamin A capsules, from acne to psoriasis to many others. It did not take too long to figure out that since this is a fat-soluble vitamin and is stored in the liver, the body could not take the amount of vitamin A necessary to treat these various conditions without creating significant side effects, from dry skin to vision problems to liver disease. Researchers tried all types of methods and formulations to try to get retinol to be stable in a cream and be able to be used on the skin, but to no avail. Finally, Dr. Al Kligman, working with many forms and derivations of vitamin A at the University of Pennsylvania, discovered that vitamin A acid (retinoic acid) was stable enough to use in creams and was active and helped clearing acne. Thus Retin-A was born. This breakthrough in the treatment of acne led to the first true cosmeceutical and opened the door to the world of cosmetic treatments of skin aging. Dr. Kligman's patient (a division of Johnson and Johnson) developed an emollient form of the cream approved by the FDA specifically for the treatment of photoaging (Renova'). However, dermatologists and their patients did not wait for the government to catch up with the desires of the baby boomers. Retin-A, and later, Renova, actually flew off the shelves to treat aging.

We have now come another few decades, and formulators have now been able to develop creams with stable forms of retinol (vitamin A). Therefore, you see the glut on the market of products containing retinol, which you never were able to obtain before. But once again, be careful. Just because there are some formulas and products on the market that have stable retinol, not all of them do and not all are equal. How in the world are you supposed to know what to do and what to use? The first source of reliable information is your dermatologist, and if that is not possible, then you should be able to rely on a well-known and trusted brand. It is unlikely that a cheap, unknown brand that says it contains retinol is going to be effective. Possibly, but not likely.

Retinol can be formulated now, but it is not easy and requires some sophisticated and expensive methods to do it right. It is also very finicky. If it is exposed to light or oxygen during manufacturing, the molecule will literally burst, and the cream will not be effective. This is often also true with products that sit on the bathroom counter and are opened repeatedly. The more the molecule is exposed to air, the less effective it is over time. Just think of what happens to a piece of apple left out on the counter overnight. This process of turning brown is scientifically known as oxidation, and it happens on some level to every cream you have every time you open the jar!

There are a number of innovative ways developed to get around this problem, and one of them that we will discuss again and again is to have a fresh dosage every time you put on your skin care product. No, you don't have to open a new jar every time. You open a new capsule every time. This innovative delivery system was developed and manufactured by Cardinal Health (now Catalent, a division of Cardinal Health) and is used for a number of products. Not only have they developed a way to deliver the product and guarantee freshness and stability every time, but even the delivery capsule is unique. The first capsules of this type were made from gelatin, an animal by-product, and the Cardinal Health ones are made of vegetable material, thus called vegicaps. These serve the same purpose as the old gelatin capsules (freshness, cleanliness, and stability) but have a big advantage in this day and time. They are totally biodegradable!

So you have a great deal of information that you can use at the cosmetic counter and the drugstore to get stable vitamin A that will perform. But what will it do? Another so what? What will it do *for me*?

Retinol or vitamin A can be viewed as the driver of the sports car that is your skin. It is in total control. The outer layer of the skin, known as the epidermis (also known as the bathtub ring or dust), is constantly turning over, making itself anew every twenty-eight days starting with plump little manufacturing plants well fed from the blood vessels just below them in the dermis to gradually flatten out and flake off. In an orderly progression, that is tightly controlled and works well until we do such stupid things such as smoking and getting out in the sun. These two things are really much more important than true aging in producing what we call "old skin." And when the outer layers of the skin become damaged, the progression of the skin cells becomes disorderly with cells going to the side instead of to the top, leaving the bottom layer too early or too late, resulting in what we see as dull, lifeless, dry, flaky, old-looking parchment; and vitamin A comes to the rescue. When active retinol, in the proper concentrations and formulation, is applied to the skin, it actually enters the nucleus or brain center of the skin cell and makes it normal again. The cells begin to slough off normally and progress to replace each other in a normal fashion, resulting in the smooth, translucent look that reminds us of baby's skin. The dead layers can come off; trapped dirt, makeup, and oil that have blocked the view of your beautiful skin begin to show through. This new skin, though, is not only pretty, but like a baby's new skin, it is sensitive and may be red and dry until you can get used to the fact that the new skin needs to be protected, moisturized and protected from the sun!

But vitamin A does even more. There is a cell in the dermis or lower part of the skin called the fibroblast. This manufacturing facility makes collagen, giving support to the skin, elastic fibers, allowing the skin to be flexible, and loves vitamin A. Fibroblasts will congregate anywhere there is vitamin A, and they will begin to increase their manufacturing abilities. This is why vitamin A helps wounds heal with little or no scars and why it helps stretch marks disappear (which really are little scars rather than just areas of the skin that have been stretched too much).

So this is why vitamin A is the skin vitamin, and every skin care regimen must contain some active form of vitamin A topically for it to be the least bit effective. Sometimes there is irritation and dryness at the beginning, but it is important not to give up and stop the vitamin A product. This can be overcome simply by discontinuing its use for a few days and restarting at every other night and building up gradually. Another useful trick to get rid of dryness is to cleanse with a mild cleanser, leave a little moisture on the face, and apply a thin film of plain petroleum jelly. If you can leave this on overnight (although it may be a bit messy), the dryness will be gone in one or two applications.

As mentioned, not all retinol products are created equal. So what brands that contain retinol can you really trust? There are many, just as there are many that you cannot. However, here's a few that you can trust that will contain active stabilized retinol that will be effective: Neutrogena Healthy Skin, RoC, Jan Marini, Peter Thomas Roth, Mary Kay, La Roche-Posay, L'Oréal, Obagi, Skinceuticals, SkinMedica, Dr. Brandt, and Murad. There are others but physicians working with chemists, who are experts in the field, formulate these, and the products have been tested and stand the test of time. They do work!

VITAMIN C

Vitamin C or ascorbic acid was first isolated and discovered in 1928 from an animal source but later found in citrus fruits. It became very important when it was determined that lack of this vitamin led to the development of scurvy, and when lemons and limes were provided to British sailors, the disease was prevented, hence the term "limies." There have been a great many studies about vitamin C over the years since its discovery and a great deal of anecdotal information that has not really been borne out by the light of scientific scrutiny such as the use of this vitamin in preventing colds. Research has certainly shown that this is a very powerful antioxidant, which means it plays a role in the protection of cells from the environment as well as from the chemicals produced as metabolism goes on. It is more in the topical use of this vitamin that uncertainty and controversy arise. This is a very unstable molecule and very difficult to formulate. Most of the early work on the use of topical vitamin C was done at Duke University and actually involved the study of the effects of vitamin C on skin or rats. When I introduced topical vitamin C a number of years ago on *Good Morning America* as a possible wrinkle reducer, the only real data that was available was that it protected rats from the long wavelength of ultraviolet light.

Many different cosmetic companies have come out with a topical vitamin C product and some with an entire line, mostly based on the story that one could tell about vitamin C, having nothing to do with topical application or any data obtained with their product. Almost all the formulations that are on the market are unstable, and it is very easy to determine if a product you are using is stable or not. When you open the jar for the first time, the cream should be bright yellow. The longer it maintains this color, the more stable it is. That still does not necessarily mean that it does anything when applied, but it probably at least has a chance. There are many other problems with topical vitamin C other than the stability issue, and there is almost no real data to support any claims made for this type of product; yet it sells, and there is a tremendous amount of anecdotal evidence that it does decrease the appearance of wrinkles, fine lines, and discolored skin due to the sun.

New technology has been developed to keep the product out of light and away from oxygen, which significantly helps in maintaining the stability of the vitamin C. This will be discussed at the end of the topical vitamin chapter.

The biggest difficulty with topical vitamin C products is trying to keep them stable and active while the consumer is using them. There are hundreds of products on the market, but the one that I have found that remains stable and effective longer than any other that I am aware of is Quintessence serum C, manufactured and distributed by International Cosmeceuticals in Miami.

VITAMIN E

Vitamin E (actually a number of different vitamins called tocopherols) is a fat-soluble vitamin as opposed to vitamin C, which is water soluble. The difference is that it does not matter how much vitamin C you ingest, it will simply go out with the urine (this, by the way, is why urine looks yellow when you take vitamins); vitamin E and other fat-soluble vitamins are stored in the liver and can build up to excess, causing some medical problems. Other fat-soluble vitamins are A, D, and K.

It is thought that when ingested, vitamin E is most important in aiding vitamin C in its antioxidant activity. It almost wraps around the vitamin C, aiding it and protecting it. However, topically, it has not been shown to have any activity at all. In formulations, it is usually listed far down the line of ingredients and is merely there in very small amounts, simply for marketing. They can state that the product contains vitamin E because consumers believe it actually does do something when applied to the skin.

As far as applying pure vitamin E from the capsule goes, there has never been any data that this does anything at all. For years, plastic surgeons have and still often recommend patients to apply it to surgical sites after surgery to prevent and reduce scars when present. This has no more effect than applying any other oily substance, be it motor oil, vegetable oil, etc. No effect at all except now you have an oily scar.

VITAMIN K

*V*itamin K has a very interesting history. It was first discovered in 1929 near Germany and was named this because it was found to aid in coagulation and named the *koagulation* vitamin. It plays a vital role in the ability of the body to make many of the factors that aid in clotting to keep us from bleeding to death when we get a cut or a scrape. Its sources are green leafy vegetables such as kale, and it is also manufactured by bacteria in the human gastrointestinal tract.

Since a newborn has no bacteria in the GI tract and obviously has not eaten any green leafy vegetables, every baby born in the most civilized countries is given a shot of vitamin K. Vitamin K plays a very vital role in our lives because without it, it would not be possible to make the various clotting factors in the liver that are necessary to keep us from bleeding to death from even a minor traumatic incident. Vitamin K is also very important as a drug when given systemically in case of accidental or intentional overdose of aspirin, too much blood thinners, or even accidental ingestion of rat poison; so it is vital in every emergency room! But what about topical vitamin K, the vitamin applied to the skin?

In the early 1990s, treatment for sun-damaged or aging skin was beginning to appear on the scene, obviously spearheaded by Retin-A as discussed before. We could treat many of the manifestations of sun-damaged or aging skin, but one disconcerting problem defied treatment. Neither Retin-A nor the new (at the time) alpha hydroxy acid such as glycolic acid, had much, if any, effect on the bruising that occurred when older individuals just barely tapped their hand. Large, ugly bruises would appear from the minor trauma and last for weeks. This is a problem I started to look at, and I tried many topical agents, some on the market, some still in research, and some just out of desperation. As it turned out, topical vitamin K not only made the bruises go away faster (actually twice as fast) but also kept bruises from occurring when applied on a regular basis to these particularly thin-skinned individuals.

This research formed the basis of what became a phenomenon over the next decade as it was shown that topical vitamin K would make any type of bruise go away faster, and then research at some of the most respected laser centers in the United States demonstrated that it made the bruising and redness from laser treatments disappear faster and could even prevent problems when used prior to treatment. More and more research by dermatologists, plastic surgeons, and aestheticians led to the use of topical vitamin K in the prevention of bruises from surgery of all types and even blood drawing. One of the interesting uses that came to the fore and was proven by a great deal of research was the use of topical vitamin K, particularly when combined with topical vitamin A to decrease the appearance of dark circles under the eyes. This is currently the most common use for topical vitamin K, although it is beginning to be used to lighten other pigment problems in the skin as well.

It should be noted that the topical application of vitamin K does not work through the liver, does not affect the clotting mechanism in healthy people or those on blood thinners, and although the mechanism of action is quite complicated, has been worked out by a researcher from Ukraine, showing the complete pathway.

So we have looked at most of the true vitamins and how they might or might not be used as topical agents for the treatment of the aging skin, but the delivery, i.e., of how the vitamin actually gets from the container to your skin and then through your skin is just as important as the vitamins themselves, and research has kept up with this aspect of treatment as well. No longer do you have to have a bunch of jars and bottles sitting around the bathroom, exposed to light, air, and most importantly, your finger and with the possibility of mixing them together.

It is a bit complicated and beyond the scope of this book to describe the various methods that are used to make certain that products get into the skin because after all, the main purpose of skin is to keep things out (a barrier between the world and the inside of the body), and it does a very good job. However, one innovation that keeps product fresh, stable, and ready for use for years is the so-called vegicap that was developed by Cardinal Health, a company with offices around the world. The vegicap is like a capsule, but there is a small and a large end. Twist off the small end and inside is a topical agent that is manufactured in the correct dose for the use of that product, and the product is fresh and has not been exposed to air or light, which will decompose many skin products, and does not have contamination from your fingers. Additionally, this unique container is made from vegetable material rather than animal material and is totally biodegradable. Many products on the market in the cosmetic and cosmeceutical industries use this new method of keeping products fresh and ready for use.

Regardless of what type of delivery system or innovative container is used for a product, it does not make any difference if the product itself is not efficacious. We have mentioned a few things that we know do work—Retin-A, vitamin K, and some of the acids that are used to peel the skin and even constitute a main ingredient in entire skin-care lines such as glycolic acid. However, how do products and services and even entire programs for beauty and longevity get to the market and become highly successful? Three words—marketing, marketing, and marketing. There are so many baby boomers, and almost everyone wants to be young and beautiful, so we are back to the beginning of the cosmetic industry—hope in a jar or a website or a book. I do not understand why a doctor and his miraculous patient appear on TV, tell us she went on his program, and in five days, all her wrinkles were gone. She felt years younger, and everything is wonderful. Why in the world would anyone think we would believe such garbage? Even a face-lift takes more than five days to heal and still will not give everything that these particular doctors promise.

When we get into specifics of what really has no effect on the skin despite outrageous claims, things get a little complicated. Some of the problem is that there are things that work when taken or have been shown to be effective in the laboratory but that has very little, if anything, to do with whether or not something will be effective when it is put into a formulation, applied to the skin, and then have to get into the skin and be effective. When one looks at the size of some of the molecules that manufacturers claim effective, it seems as if they have figured out a way to get the Empire State Building to go through the eye of a needle.

All of us want to believe so hard that things work, that they will do what the doctor or the company say they will, and we will be beautiful, healthy, and live happily ever after. I did a little research study a number of years ago. As a rather well-respected and well-known cosmetic dermatologist with a large clinical practice, I had many patients who believed in me. If I said it was so, it was so. I asked twenty women to evaluate a new cream that I had invented that I was calling "Miracle Cream." They were to apply it to their hands and thighs for a period of eight weeks and come in every two weeks for pictures that I was going to use in marketing the product. I told them I had already done the research and I wanted their valued opinion as to how much a fair price for a small jar of the cream was—twenty-five, fifty, or one hundred dollars. A few said one hundred, no one said twenty-five, and the great majority said they were willing to pay fifty dollars for this miraculous antiaging product that I had invented. The only problem was that there was nothing in the cream, just a moisturizer without any type of active ingredient. I point this out not because I think people are stupid and certainly not my patients. What this shows is the intense desire for something to work, and if you have faith in the inventor or doctor or company or spokesperson that transfers directly to the product, it has to work; and when you look in the mirror, you see the emperor's new clothes. You see what you want to see.

ALPHA HYDROXY ACIDS

This group of chemicals derives from the parent molecule, acetic acid or vinegar. Many of them occur naturally in food, especially fruit, and therefore, they are often referred to as fruit acids. Glycolic acid occurs in sugar cane, lactic in milk, tartaric in grapes, citric in limes and lemons, butyric in butter, etc. Although these all occur naturally, the products that are on the cosmetic market do not contain derivatives of the natural substance but are manufactured by chemical companies. The most important ones that have been actually used over the centuries are glycolic, lactic, tartaric, and citric. Cleopatra supposedly took advantage of the lactic acid in sour milk and bathed in it to get her skin soft and smooth, taking advantage of the natural ability of the lactic acid to moisturize the skin. Ancient Greeks would take the sludge out of the bottom of the wine vat to perform chemical peels to make the skin smoother, using the concentrated tartaric acid at the bottom after fermentation. (If you have ever drunk grappa, which is concentrated wine like this and is full of tartaric acid, you know how strong it can really be.). Citric acid, of course, occurs in its natural state in lemons and limes and has been used for centuries to bleach the skin.

There are myriads of products now on the market that utilize some form of alpha hydroxy acids. There are chemical peels available to physicians and aestheticians that contain tartaric acid, some with citric acid and some with other less common forms of alpha hydroxy acids such as mandelic acid. Moisturizers often contain lactic acid, but the most commonly used member of this group of compounds is glycolic acid. It has been used to manufacture chemical peeling products for both physicians and aestheticians with the physician product being stronger and will penetrate deeper than that of the aesthetician. Now there are also hundreds of products with glycolic acid on the market. As mentioned, this is certainly because it is the easiest and simplest of these compounds to work with. However, it is a very effective agent. Glycolic acid in products performs a number of functions. Glycolic acid loosens the attachments between the cells of the outer layer of skin, removing the dead layers, giving the skin a smoother and shinier appearance. Additionally, glycolic acid allows greater penetration of other products that are used in conjunction with it. This means, for example, that using a glycolic acid cleanser and moisturizer while also using retinol will increase the penetration of the retinol, and it will therefore be more effective. It has also been shown recently that glycolic acid does stimulate new formation of collagen and therefore does have a positive effect on the reduction of the appearance of fine lines and wrinkles. As with all aspects of cosmetics, beware! Just because this is a popular ingredient and is fairly easy to work with does not mean all products are equal. Use a brand developed by a dermatologist or one that you know you can trust due to the reputation—Avon, Mary Kay, Neutrogena, etc.

BETA HYDROXY ACIDS

This group is obviously quite similar to the alpha hydroxy acids with just a little change in the chemistry. The main one that is used in cosmetic and cosmeceutical preparations is salicylic acid. This chemical has a number of interesting uses. It is found in both cosmetic and prescription strengths in topical products for moisturizing severely dry skin and even in high doses to treat plantar warts and thick heels.

In lower concentrations, it is also very useful in acne preparations as it is one of the most effective agents to loosen the plug in the oil gland that is the cause of acne. Additionally, it is used in dermatologists' offices and in medical spas in various concentrations as a chemical peel, primarily to treat acne, and is especially beneficial in improving the appearance of blackheads.

POLYHYDROXY ACIDS

This term recently appeared in the medical literature and in beauty products but is really more of a marketing ploy than a new phenomenon. They are combinations of hydroxyl acids and do not provide significantly greater benefit to the skin.

SUNSCREENS

The FDA regulates sunscreens as over-the-counter drugs. That means that there is a written monograph that all companies that manufacture a sunscreen must follow. This contains things such as ingredients that are allowed, what you can and cannot say about the product, how the labeling is to be done, even the size of the lettering on the label. This sounds great, but the FDA really does not do a very good job in either directing what is done or policing it. A new monograph proposing changes in the way sunscreens are labeled that would significantly benefit the consumer was developed by the FDA in 1999, but the agency still has not followed through on it. There is some current activity that shows that they may actually be moving on this now.

The concept that the sun was actually harmful to the skin, and we should protect ourselves from it never occurred to the baby boomers as we were growing up. When we were lucky enough to get to a pool or a beach, we would do everything we could to get as much sun and obtain that healthy glow. This phenomenon actually came to the forefront after the Great Depression. If you go back in history, whether the 1920s or Ancient Rome, the whiter the skin was, the more there was an indication that you were in the upper class. Only farmers and laborers got tanned, brown skin and not wealthy upper class. This changed when Americans began working shorter hours and had more leisure time to spend outdoors—golfing, boating, or whatever. Now men of leisure got tans and so did the wives.

Of course, dermatologists have known for a long time that the sun causes skin cancer as well as a myriad of other diseases and problems. Therefore, sunscreens began to appear in the market to prevent sunburn and to help prevent skin cancer as early as the 1960s. Prior to that time, if anyone wanted to prevent sunburn, they would usually apply zinc oxide. The first sunscreens on the market that were not just opaque creams contained para-aminobenzoic acid (PABA). PABA was effective in preventing the short wavelength ultraviolet rays from harming the skin and therefore preventing sunburns. However, after some period of time they were used, it became apparent that there was some significant degree of allergy associated with this particular chemical. So the search was on for more effective and safer agents to use on the skin as sunscreens and sunblocks.

It took some time, but many agents have been developed and used in sunscreens that are approved by the FDA that are both safe and effective. There are those that prevent the absorption of UVB (mostly chemical blocks) and those that block UVA (both chemical and physical). A chemical block reacts with an entity in the skin to prevent the energy from getting in, whereas a physical block acts like a miniature umbrella. That is why many of the agents contain micronized zinc oxide or something of the sort.

A few things should be pointed out about sunscreens. In the United States, a sunscreen has an SPF rating on the label. SPF stands for "sun protection factor" and refers to the degree to which the agent protects you from burning in terms of time. If you burn in ten minutes, then applying a sunscreen with an SPF 15 theoretically will allow you to stay out in the sun without burning for 150 minutes. This is not completely true for a number of reasons. First, the SPF of a product is tested in the laboratory under controlled conditions and with the use of controlled amount of product. In the real world, people do not all apply the same amount of product, nor do they apply it properly, and one must take into account the effects of wind, perspiration, getting into the pool or ocean, etc. Sunscreen should be applied evenly over the surface of the skin at least thirty minutes prior to going outside and reapplying every hour or so unless perspiration is excessive or you go into the water, in which case you will need to apply it more often. You should use an amount equal to a teaspoon for the face, each arm and leg, and twice that amount for the front of the torso and the same for the back. Hats certainly do help, and now there is actually clothing being manufactured with SPF built right into the fabric. Additionally, do not forget the primary cause of cataracts is the UVA spectrum of light, so always wear sunglasses with UVA protective lenses when you are outside.

The discussion of products, whether they be cosmetics, cosmeceuticals or over-the-counter drugs like sunscreens, should not end without a significant warning to you. I have worked with a number of drug, cosmetic, and cosmeceutical companies, and they certainly vary as to their attention to detail and desire to be certain that products are both effective and safe. One of the most diligent companies I have encountered is Johnson and Johnson. A number of years ago, I worked with one of the Johnson and Johnson companies (there are hundreds of them) to develop a skin-care line based on glycolic acid. There was not only attention to making certain that all the products were safe and effective, but great care was taken to make sure that absolutely every base was covered. Was the packaging safe? Was the ink in the packaging safe? Would it be possible to have any interaction with the product and the packaging that would damage the product? This went on and on for months and paid off in a line that was launched and became very successful.

On the other hand, I worked with a small cosmetics company to advise them on product development and how to comply with FDA regulations on claims and labeling. I found out pretty quickly that the company was much more interested in stating that they had a dermatologist as a consultant than they were at taking any advice. The first thing I noticed was that the labeling had print that was too small. Yes, the FDA regulates the size of the font on a label to be certain that it could easily be read. I pointed this out and was subsequently ignored. Then I asked about how they know that their products were effective and that they were safe. The answer was that they sell, and they did not have many returns, so they must be both safe and effective. No clinical trials. No allergy or safety testing. No testing of the formulations. Nothing. And that, unfortunately, is the way business is done in much of the cosmetic industry but not all. So once again, choose carefully, be a wise consumer, and ask questions.

THE MINI LIFT

O ver the last few decades, a new form of treatment for the gravity factor or falling off face has come to the fore. It goes by many names—mini lift, curl lift, string lift, etc. Essentially, these are all procedures that purport to lift the skin of the face and/or neck by inserting suture material through small openings in the scalp or face area, pulling up the skin, and resulting in a refreshed, youthful appearance without having to undergo general anesthesia or extensive surgery. So what is the story?

First, it depends on what they promise. Certainly, there can be some benefit achieved from such a procedure; however, many times, patients are told the results will last for five years or more, and I simply have not seen that to be the case. Additionally, there are so many questions that you need to ask before you submit to a procedure such as this.

Where is the location they intend for the procedure? In a sterile operating room, a clean room, or just a treatment room? Is it in a doctor's office, a hospital, or a spa? Who is going to do it? Is that person board certified in a specialty that deals with this type of procedure? How many has the doctor done, and who trained the doctor? What side effects have occurred, and how has the staff handled these?

There have been reports of side effects such as infection, unevenness, failure, etc. as high as 30 percent, and that is unacceptable for any procedure. In addition, despite what is promised by some locations, these will not last for five years even in the most experienced hands. From what I have seen, the results last about a year. However, there are many instances of the suture material having to be removed because of foreign body reactions or other reasons that never allow any longevity to the procedure. (Foreign body reactions occur because of the facial hair that may get trapped in the area of the incision and suturing.)

One of the problems with this procedure is that there are so many variations, and some have been presented at medical meetings and some have been published in the medical literature and some have not. There is no way that one can really discern whether they ought to get involved with such a procedure. Probably the best way to at least begin to make an informed intelligent decision is that if the procedure is done in a dermatologist's or plastic surgeon's office, and you can be shown results obtained by that doctor that you think is reasonable; then you may proceed, but never let someone who is a hired doctor in one of these medical spas perform this type of procedure on you. If you really need a face-lift, get a face-lift!

MESOTHERAPY

Mesotherapy is a procedure that is gaining some prominence outside the United States and beginning to catch on a little in this country. It is promoted under various names, from mesotherapy to lipodissolve to many other monikers. It is not well thought of in most surgical and cosmetic circles, and there are very few, if any, controlled studies as to what this procedure actually does and what the possible side effects and other consequences may be.

Basically, a concoction of substances such as chemicals to dissolve fat, vitamins, hormones, and many other substances are injected into the fat through a small needle. The procedure is somewhat uncomfortable but not painful, and some physicians have obtained significant reduction in fat and some sculpting of the body. One of the problems is that there is no standard cocktail of what is injected and no controlled studies of any significance as to what should or should not be injected. It has also been advertised to remove cellulite, which it does not do, and the side effects are rarely found in any of the print advertising or marketing. Of course, infection can occur with any procedure, and that includes this one. Bruising is not unusual, and at this point, there appear to be no significant side effects other than not get the results that are advertised.

One of the constituents that is always in the injection mixture is phosphatidylcholine, which is, by no means, a benign drug. This can cause a great deal of inflammation, irritation, and swelling wherever it is injected. Even Brazil, where drug approvals are significantly less strict than the United States and where beautiful bodies are the norm and always desired, this drug has been banned.

The procedure is not new; this multiple injection technique was actually developed in France in the 1950s and has some popularity among doctors particularly in Europe. In the United States, there is only a small fraction of doctors performing this procedure, and it is certainly a controversial procedure. At this time, it is best to simply avoid these procedures advertised as mesotherapy, lipodissolve, etc.

BOTOX

One of the greatest advances in the treatment of the aging baby boomer's face and, indeed, one of the main reasons that you are even reading this book is the advent of Botox. I have already touched on this previously but not really discussing how this evolved, why it did, and what it can and cannot do.

It is true that Botox stands for botulinum toxin, but it is not really an injection of botulism at all. The analogy to penicillin is sensible in that penicillin is derived from a mold, but when you get a shot of penicillin, you are not getting an injection of the mold. The same holds true for this material. Botox and the other botulinum toxin derivatives that are on the market are from the botulinum organism, but you are not getting an injection of botulism or even the pure toxin. In actuality, we are using millionths of the amount necessary to even begin to induce any type of problem throughout the body.

But how did this even get started anyway? The use of this material was well known in the '70s for military use, and in the 1980s, it began to be used as approved by the FDA for blepharospasm (inability to control eye blinking) and other eye problems. One of the prominent ophthalmologists in Vancouver noticed that when she was injecting her patients for these types of problems, the lines around the eyes were going away. It just happens that her husband is a dermatologist, and the two of them developed the technique for treating not only the lines around the eyes but also the frown lines as well.

Even though the consensus is that Botox injections are new, having been around for only a few years, in actuality, a number of doctors have been using it for cosmetic purposes since the late 1980s. Clinical trials were finally performed, and the injections were approved by the FDA for treating the frown line in 2003. That is when advertising and marketing for the cosmetic use began, and that is when it became such a famous procedure.

How does it actually work? One needs to understand that botulinum injections (whether Botox or Dysport or Xeomin or one of the other materials of this nature around the world) do not treat lines. This is not a filling material. Filling materials treat lines; botulinum treats muscles

46

that cause the lines. That is why it can only be used in certain areas. Muscles that cause lines by constant pulling have to be isolated and injected. It is easy to isolate the three muscles that cause the frown line to occur, whereas it is very difficult to isolate muscles that could cause the smile lines from the corner of the nose to the corner of the mouth. Once the muscles are able to be isolated, the injections can be performed; but again, one must keep in mind that since the cause of the lines and not the lines are being injected, it takes time for the effect to occur. Generally, it takes at least three to five days for the injections to begin to work, seven to ten days to reach its peak, and then the effect will last for a number of months, depending on the site of the injection and skill of the injector. If done properly, there should be very little, if any, pain and minimal bruising with the injections. Following the injections, you should not lie flat for eight hours, should not massage the area, and should not bend over and pick up heavy objects. Application of topical vitamin K cream will reduce any tendency of bruising and decrease the appearance of the tiny needle marks. Ice also helps in this capacity. Additionally, to ensure the procedure works as quickly as possible, try to use the muscles that were injected frequently during the day.

Although, the only area approved by the FDA for injection of Botox is the frown line, many other areas are frequently injected, and more and more uses are being found for this versatile substance every day. The three most common areas that are treated are the frown line, the crow's feet around the eyes, and the forehead lines. Botox can also be used successfully under the eyes by experienced injectors for the fine lines in that area, to raise the nasal tip, to soften the bunny lines at the bridge of the nose, to soften a harsh-appearing chin, soften the neck lines, decrease the appearance of the neck bands and lift the face, decrease the appearance of the crinkle lines of the décolleté and many uses are added daily. There are even procedures to taper the face from a square appearance to an oval one and, believe it or not, even to taper the appearance of so-called piano legs.

There will, of course, be more and more procedures and uses for this material in the future, but the main thing to remember is to make certain that the doctor (and it should be a doctor) has the basic understanding of how to use the material and the experience that will allow him to take on a new procedure *on your body.*

FILLING MATERIALS

Most of you who have been around for some time knowing about this industry probably think of this as collagen injections since collagen was the first material developed to be injected to improve the appearance of lines and wrinkles. But we have come a great distance since then. Collagen injections, which were derived from cowhide, were approved by the FDA in 1981, and I started injecting the material almost immediately. I soon began teaching doctors in the United States how to inject the material and, up to this point, have taught doctors in fifty-one countries how to use Botox and filling materials. The advance in filling materials over the last twenty-five years is nothing short of phenomenal. By the year 2000, there were almost two hundred agents available for use around the world, and now there are over three hundred. Only about twenty are approved by the FDA for use in this country.

The most popular filling material at this point in time is the hyaluronic acid products. Collagen injections, which were derived from cowhide, required a skin test in the arm prior to being injected in the face because of the possibility of allergy. As a matter of fact, most knowledgeable physicians performed two skin tests instead of one before injecting the face because of the research that I did, showing decrease in allergic reactions with two skin tests instead of one. Hyaluronic acid is not a protein and is the same molecule in every species, so it does not require skin testing prior to use. This is a big advantage since there should be no allergic reaction to the material, and there is no waiting to have the procedure done. Going to the White House tomorrow and want to look better? No problem!

Although there are probably hundreds of hyaluronic acid products on the market around the world, at the moment, there are only few that are far and above the best of the bunch. Juvederm has been shown to be the smoothest, longest lasting and least uncomfortable to have injected of the available products in the United States. There are at the moment two forms—Juvéderm Ultra, which is used for most of the work that is done with fillers, and Juvederm Ultra Plus, which is used for deeper work and can be used in the lips. There is also a product meant to be used for fine lines around the eyes and lips but is not yet FDA approved.

Hyaluronic acid products remain the most popular of the available filling materials because they provide such smooth results. It should be noted here that hyaluronic acid is a normal constituent of the skin and accounts for the turgidity and smoothness of a baby's face. Essentially, hyaluronic acid is a great trapper of water, and that is not only why it adds so much substance to the young face, but it is also why it gives such a smooth result when injected. It is also why our eyes stay moist and why our joints glide over each other. But they are not the only ones approved for use in the United States. Three others deserve to be mentioned: Sculptra, Bellafil, and Radiesse. Sculptra is a filling material that is also naturally occurring, and once injected, it degrades over time to lactic acid, which is the acid in milk. It has been shown to induce new collagen formation so that results are long lasting (over one and a half years), although it is not very popular with the doctors injecting filling materials.

Bellafil is an interesting material and is in somewhat limited use in this country. It was recently approved by the FDA, which surprised me as it is a permanent filler, and I thought the FDA would never approve a permanent filling material. It contains two components: the first is bovine solution (similar to the old collagen injections) and the second is a suspension of beads made of plexiglass. The bovine solution produces the initial correction and places the plexiglass in the area, which attracts ingrowth of new collagen fibers. The plexiglass is permanent and remains in the area. In my view, this is not a good idea, placing a material into the skin that remains forever. In my opinion, there are many reasons, but basically, two will suffice. First is that the skin changes, and the filling material may not change with it. Much more important is the fact that everyone makes a mistake, and if a mistake is made with a permanent filler, the results may be very unpleasant. I am aware of patients who had surgery to have the material removed when an adverse event occurred. Even though it is tempting to think that if you have this injected, you will not need more injections in the future, and it sounds like a good idea, it is simply foolish. You will not save any money, and it will not be worth it if you end up with a deformity that will require surgery to repair.

At the moment, these are the filling materials that are approved by the FDA for use in the United States: Zyderm and Zyplast (cow collagen), Cosmoderm and Cosmoplast (human collagen), Restylane,

Perlane, Hylaform, Hylaform Plus, Juvéderm Ultra, Juvéderm Ultra Plus, Captique (hyaluronic acid products), Sculptra (polymer of lactic acid), Artefill (permanent with plexiglass beads), and Radiesse (gel with degradable polymer). However, there are hundreds more on the market around the world, some of which will be approved eventually in the United States and some won't. Also, you travel a great deal and may want to get some material injected that is not yet approved in this country. If you are thinking about this, the best way to find out exactly what is going on with the product is to find out who the manufacturer is, and go to that company's website to get the information, and then check out the doctor who is treating you and *make sure he is a doctor!* Then you may want to proceed. There are actually many excellent products around the world that have not yet made it to this country and some who do not intend to enter this market because of the expense and time dealing with the FDA. Just do your homework.

What are the best materials for filling and contouring the face? I have already stressed that you never should allow anyone to inject a filler with a permanent material such as silicone or Artefill. But what are the best? Currently, there are not a great number available in the United States, but there are hundreds around the world, and some of you may actually be getting treatments outside the United States. When and if you do, you must be careful not to let anyone inject materials that are permanent (even though they may be said to be semipermanent), for example, Dermalive and Dermadeep, which are available in Canada and some other countries.

Although, collagen injections started the treatment of lines, wrinkles, and scars over twenty-five years ago, they are not in vogue any longer. However, there is one that has recently been approved by FDA, and that is Evolence, which is a pig-derived collagen and can be administered without a prior skin test. There is not a great deal of experience with this material yet, so the jury is still out as to how well it really works and how long it will last. As mentioned, the hyaluronic acid fillers are the most prevalent used in the world, including the United States at this time. There are many reasons for this. No skin test is required as there should be no allergy to this substance. It gives a long-lasting improvement without having the problems of a permanent filler, and it gives an extremely smooth appearance because of the affinity of hyaluronic acid for water, and that, of course, will produce the smoothest appearance of all. There is nothing smoother than the surface of water. In the United States, there are a few filling materials that are approved that contain hyaluronic acid—Restylane, Perlane, Juvéderm, Juvéderm Ultra, Captique, and Elevesse. There are a few nuances to each of these, and you and your physician can discuss which best filler for your particular situation is.

There are other filling materials available in the US that you may encounter. Cosmoderm and Cosmoplast, as mentioned, are human collagen and do not require a skin test; however, they are not long lasting (three to four months) fillers. Sculptra is a polymer of a natural substance (lactic acid) and is used by a number of physicians with excellent results, but this is more for producing volume correction than just treating lines and wrinkles. I personally do not use this material because of the difficulty with getting into proper solution, which has nothing to do with its efficacy.

In my opinion, the material currently on the market in the United States that is the most useful for many purposes that patient's desire are the products based on hyaluronic acid.

CHEMICAL PEELS

The use of agents applied to the skin to peel it is certainly not new. In the process of making wine in ancient Greece, the acid in the bottom of the vat after the wine was made was applied to the face to rejuvenate it. Women did not know it, but they were simply applying tartaric acid to perform a chemical peel and make the skin smoother. The concept of chemical peeling is really quite simple. The pH of the skin is 5.5. Anything that is applied to change that will injure the skin and produce wounding which will then peel and heal with improvement to the skin if done properly.

A chemical peel could be performed using alkali—lye—instead of acids, i.e., raise the pH rather than lower it. However, alkali is not controllable or predictable and can produce severe burns. So we use acid to injure the skin and produce the wounding, which then peels, and the skin should look better, smoother, etc. when all is said and done. Chemical peeling can be done by utilizing many, many acids. The stronger the acid, the greater the peeling and the better the results but the greater the chance of scarring or other side effects.

The mildest of all the chemical peels currently in use is the low-strength glycolic acid peels. I was instrumental in developing MD Formulations line and peels when I was medical director of Herald Pharmacal, and the purpose of the mild peel for the aestheticians to use was to be sure that no one could be harmed with the peel. We developed two strengths—the milder one for the aestheticians and a stronger one for physicians, but glycolic acid still is relatively mild. Glycolic acid peels are timed peels, i.e., the acid is left on the skin for a period of time, and then cool water is applied. When this is done, we say that we are neutralizing the acid, but I don't think that is really true. We are just wiping it off and cooling the skin. At any rate, this mild type of peel stings a little and may produce a bit of redness for a day or so and demonstrate very little and true peeling, but it does freshen the skin and make it feel a little smoother. Generally, these peels are done in a series of six, but the results are not dramatic. There will be very little change in fine lines and wrinkles and virtually no change in splotchiness of the skin.

Glycolic acid is the simplest of all the alpha hydroxy acids, also known as AHAs, and there are many peels derived from other acids in this group. Although all of these occur in nature, e.g., glycolic from sugar cane, mandelic from apples, and tartaric from grapes, the fruit is not the source of any of the acids used. They do occur in nature, but the ones used in medicine are manufactured by chemical companies.

Salicylic acid is a beta hydroxy acid and is frequently used especially to treat acne and complexion problems since it gets into the oil gland better than other acids and can aid in clearing the plug out of the oil gland. This peel is not a timed peel because as soon as it is applied, it turns to a powder and does not affect the skin any longer than the immediate effect. There is a strong odor of wintergreen as this is a derivative of this acid, and people who are allergic to aspirin (acetylsalicylic acid) should not have this peel done. Various strengths are used, but this still remains a relatively mild peel with redness and some scaling occurring over only a couple of days.

Although there are many mixtures of various acids and formulas that are used by dermatologists to perform chemical peeling, only a few have found their way into the armamentarium of general cosmetic use. Trichloroacetic acid is the most commonly utilized medium to deep chemical peeling agent. The concentration of the acid determines its depth, and sometimes, dermatologists apply other acids or perform procedures to make the acid penetrate deeper. Aestheticians use 10%–20% and should not use anything to enhance the penetration. Physicians use 35%–50%. This type of peel must be neutralized, and the whiteness that is seen is actually a coagulation of protein of the skin as opposed to the precipitate that occurs with salicylic acid. It is quite painful, especially in the higher concentrations. Peeling may last for weeks, and care must be taken to prevent exposure to the sun and other elements, and infection must be avoided. This peel can scar and can result in pigment problems, especially in patients with darker skin. The higher strengths (thirty-five and above) or combinations with other agents should never be done by anyone but a physician who is very knowledgeable about skin and how it heals. One of the gimmicks that has been developed is to put a chemical in to indicate pH change that occurs with the peel, and you have the so-called blue peel.

The deepest of all chemical peels is based on phenol or carbolic acid and should never be done except by a physician and under monitored conditions as this peel can affect the heart and kidneys. It is rarely performed any longer.

In the right hands and for the correct indications, chemical peels remain an effective method in combination with proper at-home care and other procedures to reverse the aging appearance.

MICRODERMABRASION

Before discussing microdermabrasion, we should address the more significantly effective procedure—dermabrasion. It is very important not to confuse the two because they are as different as night and day. Dermabrasion is a tried and true, albeit older, method of treating acne scars, acne, and photoaged skin. It was invented in the 1930s by a dermatologist, using a fast rotating wire brush to remove the outer layers of the skin and allowing the skin to heal smoother. In more recent years, rotating diamonds have been used to perform the procedure. It is very skill dependent, requires anesthesia and many hours to perform, and takes two to three weeks to heal correctly. Because of the difficulty of properly performing the procedure and getting good results and the fact that there is a great deal of blood involved during the procedure, it is no longer performed by many practitioners.

Microdermabrasion is a procedure born in the last decade that is similar to sandblasting a building. Initially, it was actually done with sand that was forced onto the skin at a very high velocity and was quite a messy procedure. Now it has undergone some improvements in that various fine particles are used to spray onto the skin in a closed system that removes them as they are applied. The question is simple: What are the benefits of microdermabrasion? The answer: not much. The removal of the very outer layers of the skin may make the skin feel smoother, may make makeup temporarily go on smoother, and may prepare the skin for other procedures, but the fact is that it is too superficial for a procedure to produce much change in the skin at all. This is truly the emperor's new clothes. You could get the same amount of benefit by rubbing a dry washcloth roughly over the face. Don't fall for paying for a series of these to try to make any difference in the way your skin looks. If microdermabrasion is done prior to a procedure or in combination, it very well may be worth it (such as combined with a light chemical peel), but as a stand-alone treatment, it is not worth what you pay for it.

LIPOSUCTION

Although liposuction in various forms has been around for centuries, its popularity waxes and wanes. There are many misconceptions regarding this procedure, and there are many new and innovative approaches to this. First and foremost, liposuction is not a treatment to cure obesity. True, it does remove fat, but it is really a form of body sculpting to change the appearance and make the body more attractive by removing or moving areas of fat, most commonly, the love handles, the chin and/or jowls, the thighs and knees, and even the arms. Some fat can be removed from the abdominal area, but to remove very large amounts of fat can be a very dangerous procedure as there can be a significant amount of blood loss, electrolyte imbalance, and the result can be shock and even death.

If you are contemplating even having small amounts of fat removed to improve your statuesque appearance, there are a number of things you must take into account. First and foremost, who is going to do this procedure? Make sure that this is not going to be done by some doctor who got bored with his or her former specialty and decided to take a weekend course in liposuction. You must have either a board-certified plastic surgeon or a board-certified dermatologist perform this type of procedure. There are some experts and many are plastic surgeons performing this, but there are some very experienced, true experts in the field of dermatology. You also need to be sure of the facility where the procedure will be done. Best is an operating room in a hospital or surgical center, but it can be done in an office operating room. *But* do your homework. Check and make sure that the facility is approved by insurance companies such as Medicare (even though insurance is not going to pay for the procedure); check as to what type of anesthesia will be used and if there will be an anesthesiologist or anesthetist present. And above all, check out the doctor—what specialty, what board certification, how many of these procedures has been done by him, and what are the results. Will he show you before and after pictures of his patients, not just pictures of what liposuction can do for someone.

There are some nuances to the story of liposuction, although it has been around off and on for centuries. First of all, there is lipotransfer or the harvesting of fat from one area of the body to enhance another area by injecting it into the donor site. This is done by a number of specialists, and some are extremely talented and get excellent results, but they are few and far between. You need to really check their credentials here, and in my opinion, this is not a procedure that should be done as a stand alone for the treatment of wrinkles and folds but only in conjunction with a liposuction procedure that is already being contemplated.

There are a number of procedures that have been attached to ordinary liposuction to supposedly make it more rapid or provide better healing or smoother results. One is ultrasonic liposuction during which ultrasound is used to break up the fat and make it easier to remove. You may find some doctors using this. It has been around for at least fifteen years or longer and probably does not offer what is promised. A much newer procedure developed by a dermatologist in New York City is laser-assisted liposuction or so-called SmartLipo. In this procedure, a laser is used to burst the fat into a liquid, and the fat is therefore easier to remove, which gives a better result and is less traumatic to the patient. If your doctor is contemplating this procedure, be sure he is experienced as this is a rather new technique, and there are only certain doctors who are real experts in this form of liposuction.

Regardless of which type of liposuction you may undergo, the skin may not snap back as much as you would like or expect and that it would lead to another procedure, removing the excess skin that is left as the support is removed. This is also true in patients who undergo significant weight loss, either through surgery or diet. The skin that has been stretched for over a long period of time simply is not that resilient.

LASERS

I will be the first to admit I am not an expert on lasers or laser therapy, so this section is going to be short, and I suggest you go to the website of American Society for Laser Medicine and Surgery and American Society for Dermatologic Surgery for up-to-date, accurate information.

Lasers are not the magic everyone thinks them to be, and just as is the case with everything else in medicine and surgery, there is an interaction between the device and the one who is operating it. First of all, lasers are very expensive and change or get updated frequently, so it is not easy for anyone to keep up with the latest innovation. Also, the companies are coming out with machines so fast, and the competition is so stiff that there is not always a great deal of research going into the new machines and new models. The most important item is the same that I have been stressing throughout this book, and that is not the machine but the person operating the machine. Every laser in every location should be operated under the eyes of an experienced dermatologist or plastic surgeon or the equivalent thereof such as oculoplastic surgeon or facial plastic surgeon. Additionally, although I have seen advertisements that the FDA has approved certain operators in certain spas, there is never any certification offered by the FDA for any person doing anything. It is true that the FDA approves the device and the claims that are made, but that is as far as it goes. Just as in anything else we have been discussing, *beware*! Do not let an aesthetician in some medspa under the direction of a general practitioner or no doctor at all perform laser treatments on you.

THERMAGE

Good news! This procedure and the company that developed it actually live up to its marketing and advertising. As you can surmise from the name of the procedure, heat is involved somehow. Thermage utilizes radio waves that penetrate the skin to the middle layer. Although heat is involved, there is a cooling unit on the tip that touches the skin, so there is not a great deal of discomfort involved. The patient should feel that something is being done, but it should not hurt. If it does, the technician should turn down the amount of energy, and if there is no sensation at all, the energy should be increased.

As skin ages, the collagen in the middle part of the skin becomes weaker. If you can imagine a spring that is tightly wound, when the spring ages, it lengthens and no longer has the support within itself. This is also true with the collagen fibers in the skin, and this is one of the reasons that skin begins to sag with age. Thermage targets this fiber and actually has two effects. It repairs the collagen fibers and tightens them. How does it do this? Essentially, it is similar to what happens when you microwave the leftover piece of roast beef to warm it up, and then it becomes so tough, you cannot eat it. It is because the energy from the microwave while heating also shortened and tightened the fibers. Thermage does not use microwaves, but the concept is similar.

Another way that Thermage can improve the appearance of the skin is that it is inducing a wound in the skin from the heat, and anytime this occurs, skin heals and replaces the old collagen with new. So Thermage actually repairs the old collagen and induces new collagen formation.

Thermage has been used for some time in tightening the skin of the face and neck to give somewhat of a lift. It has more recently been used to tighten the skin of the arms (so-called bingo wings), the thighs, especially where baggy skin comes over the knees, and more recently, the eyelids and the hands. I have seen excellent results with this technique, but again, choose carefully. Be certain that the technician is well trained and the facility is well managed.

Thermage can be performed as a stand-alone therapy but works much more efficiently when combined with other therapies and topical agents. One must keep in mind that Thermage does not provide the instant gratification of filling materials. It takes time for the collagen to be repaired and new collagen to form. There will be nothing noticeable for a number of weeks, but then slowly over a period of up to six months, improvement will be obvious. The procedure can be repeated but not until the patient waits at least six months. There is a great deal of controversy and some misinformation as to how long the results from Thermage actually last. Some clinicians have told patients that the results last for five years, but the process has not even been in existence that long. From what I have seen, you should be able to count on a couple of years of results from the single treatment as this is not a series of treatments but only one.

TANNING BEDS

O ver the centuries, while attempting to improve the appearance of skin and enhance beauty, many things have been invented. The most dangerous one ever invented is the tanning bed. The idea, of course, is simple and straightforward. Most people do not live in Southern California or Miami, and they wanted to keep that healthy glow that was obtained in the summer at the beach. Nothing could be more ludicrous. That golden glow is not the least bit healthy, but marketing and advertising are strong incentives, and the tanning bed industry has spent millions of dollars convincing Americans that the tanning beds are safe and can make you beautiful and healthy. Nothing, nothing could be farther from the truth.

What is a tanning bed anyway? I have already discussed the fact that the sun emits various wavelengths of light and that the tanning spectrum or long wavelength is UVA. Since UVB is known as the burning spectrum, tanning beds were developed that put out intense UVA rays to tan but supposedly not burn.

There are many issues regarding tanning beds. Basically, when all the information is put together the message is "stay away!" The first issue is that even if by some stretch of the imagination, we assume they are safe. There is no real FDA regulation and no state guidelines that are in place and must be followed. If you own a gas station and you want to put in a tanning bed, then you certainly may, and the likelihood that any agency—state, federal, or local—will ever come by to check things out approaches zero. When a tanning bed is purchased, guidelines are included that go over the safety aspects such as making certain individuals wear goggles, checking on various medicines, and how to check the lights to be sure that they are emitting light properly, but these guidelines are rarely followed.

Even if every guideline is followed, there are still a myriad of issues with these tanning beds. They mostly emit UVA, the tanning spectrum, although some also emit UVB, the burning spectrum, to make their action much faster. Remember, even though UVB causes sunburn and is a direct cause of basal cell carcinoma, the most common type of skin cancer, UVA causes melanoma, which is the most dangerous form of skin cancer and also penetrates much deeper than UVB and is the main factor in aging of the skin. UVA is also the wavelength of sunlight that causes cataracts. Additionally, the light can react with many agents that are ingested or applied to the skin to cause severe rashes or burning—tetracycline antibiotics, diabetes medicine, high blood pressure medicine, psychiatric drugs, perfumes, antibacterial soap, and many, many other substances.

Usually, the beds are not properly cleaned and cared for, and the lights are almost never tested to be certain that they are functioning properly. In addition to all these things that tanning beds cause or contribute, the worst may be something that you've never heard of and that is that there is a cell in the skin called a Langerhans cell. It is the function of this cell to provide the first line of defense against infections, particularly viruses such as the herpes virus and HIV. UVA from the tanning bed destroys this cell, decreasing your immunity and making you more vulnerable to these and other infections.

Most of the attendees of such places as tanning salons are usually young women who believe that they are invincible and nothing bad will happen to them, but the effects of the tanning bed are cumulative and never go away. These young ladies will also be the ones to tell you that they are getting a base for their tan so that when they go to the beach, they won't burn. Unfortunately, the tanning provides no protection from the sun. The only point left is for them to claim that they get that healthy glow that is so popular. Well, it is now becoming popular not to be tanned just as it is becoming popular not to smoke, and that is very welcome news.

Even more disturbing is that recently, the tanning bed industry has launched a media blitz to inform the public that tanning beds are safe and that dermatologists warnings regarding all the dangers are self-serving. Let's look at their claims: First of all, they state that UVA is completely safe since it will not burn. As I have pointed out, it is true that the burning spectrum of sunlight is UVB (the shorter wavelength); but it is certainly possible to be burned from UVA, and it is more likely that a burn will occur from the intense UVA present in tanning beds than from actual exposure to the sun, and this type of burn can be extremely severe since this wavelength of light penetrates much deeper than the other. I have already pointed out that there is a plethora of evidence to support the fact that tanning beds definitely contribute to aging, and there is no doubt that they contribute to the development of malignant melanoma, the deadliest form of skin cancer and one of the few types of cancers in which the incidence continues to rise.

But the linchpin of the tanning bed industry's media campaign to inform the public of the true benefits of tanning beds is the constant haranguing that tanning beds keep individuals from becoming vitamin D deficient. This is a totally ludicrous claim on many fronts. It is true that the nutritional status of Americans is not that great; however, there has not been demonstrated a case of rickets in this country in a very long time. Rickets is the disease that results from a deficiency of vitamin D. This industry, however, is attempting to convince the public that without the tanning bed, you may become vitamin D deficient, and this will lead to soft bones, broken hips, etc. This is ludicrous and false too.

There is some controversy as to whether or not vitamin D is actually a vitamin at all since it is manufactured in the skin from a precursor from cholesterol. Some scientists actually classify it as a hormone, but that is a moot point. The main point of discussion here is the fact that vitamin D is manufactured from the precursor in the skin upon exposure to ultraviolet light, *but it is exposure to UVB* that is necessary for this chemical transformation to occur, and the tanning beds are basically UVA. This wavelength of light plays no role in manufacturing vitamin D in the skin, so the entire premise of the tanning bed lobby does not make any sense at all. They are dangerous; they provide no benefit of any sort. They are not regulated, and the only thing to do is to stay away from them. All of us get enough, incidental sun exposure regardless of where we live and regardless of the time of year to avoid any problems with vitamin D deficiency.

REGULATIONS

This is a good jump-off point to begin a discussion of how all these myriads of products that are available to you are regulated. True, every country has its own regulatory system; and it is rare to even find two that match, but let's look at the United States. Regardless of where a product is made or who makes it anywhere in the world, if it comes into the United States for sale, it will be regulated by the US law.

Basically, all of what has gone until recently in the cosmetic industry is regulated by the Cosmetics, Drug, and Toiletries Act of 1938. This law was passed because there were so many products being sold without any regulation at all, and all types of claims were being made. Essentially, the law states that a cosmetic doesn't really do anything. It has no action and no interaction with the body, in this instance, the skin. It only adorns, something that is applied to the skin that improves its appearance but has no effect on the way the skin behaves. Drugs, on the other hand, interact with the skin and have an effect that can be measured and proven.

Over the last few decades, it has become increasingly obvious that there are products, which have been developed and sold without a prescription and without seeing any doctor, that are applied to the skin and actually make a difference. These are called cosmeceuticals, and even though the FDA does not recognize the term, it does have meaning to those in the cosmetic, dermatologic, and beauty industry. It is ridiculous for anything to be regulated by a law that is almost one hundred years old and really has very little meaning or relevance to the real world.

I have worked with the FDA on a number of occasions with drugs, devices, (filling materials are regulated as devices just as are wheel chairs, canes, and IV poles) and biologics (Botox is a biologic since it is derived from a bacterium). I have to say that they are a strange group with which to work. You never know what they are thinking or what they are going to do, and their rules seem to change with the wind. As can be seen from the various problems and recalls that have been evident over the recent years and the publicity of withholding needed drugs for terminally ill patients, there is room for a lot of improvement in this agency.

I was amazed that it took so long for the agency to approve other botulinum A toxins (Dysport and Xeomin), and products for very fine line injections such as Restylane Fine Lines or Touch, which is used all over the world with great success and is needed as part of the armamentarium that should be made available to cosmetic surgeons and physicians are not yet approved for use in the US. Additionally, much to my shock, the agency approved a permanent filling material that is definitely going to cause trouble and significant side effects. It is not only that the material is permanent, which is problem enough, but the doctors who use the product are not at all skilled in the art and science of soft tissue augmentation and will be obtaining devastating results, which may very well eventuate in the patient having to have surgical correction of the problem created. In my opinion, this permanent filler will be off the market in the US in a few years. It simply is too dangerous for general use, especially in the hands of amateur injectors.

There are many hundreds of filling materials available throughout the world, and most of them are not approved by the FDA for use in this country. It is not that they are not safe or effective—because most of them are—but that companies are often hesitant to go to the FDA to get a product approved because of both the lengthy process (years) and the tremendous amount of money it takes to get through the approval process.

Since many of you travel throughout the world, it is certainly within the realm of possibility that you would desire a procedure to be performed somewhere outside this country with a filling material you are not familiar with. Just ask the doctor about it, his experience with it just like you would in this country, and also check the doctor out. He earned his reputation there just as the doctors in the United States.

REGULATION OF PHYSICIANS AND PROCEDURES

Just as there are regulations in the United States by FDA and other bodies and there are regulations for cosmetics and drugs throughout the world, more scrutiny is beginning to be applied to physicians themselves and the procedures that are performed all over the world . There are a myriad of types of physicians getting into the world of cosmetic surgery and aesthetic medicine, and I have touched on that in many areas of this book already. Here, I am not going to go into great detail about the physicians who are performing procedures but would like to address the role of governmental agencies and various procedures being performed.

First, let's look at what the governments are doing and what they need to do. I have never been a big fan of any interference by the government in any of my affairs; however, there comes a time when something has to be done to protect the public (in this instance, patients) from forces which seem to be spiraling out of control. There are simply too many unqualified doctors and nondoctors performing cosmetic procedures and practicing aesthetic medicine. Again and again, in this book, I have emphasized the training necessary to be able to perform the minimum basic noninvasive procedures such as Botox injections, filling materials, and some types of chemical peels. Some of the so-called noncore physicians do take courses that are intense and can become certified and qualified to perform these procedures, but many doctors are not bothering to become properly trained because these procedures are so simple. But they are not so simple. Not only that things can, do, and will go wrong; and when things go wrong, the doctor who performed the procedure needs to know how to take care of the patient after the procedure, no matter what happens. Some of the doctors are actually going online and getting training from a website and then receive a certificate stating that they are qualified. Some are trained to become experts in weekend courses. Some are trained by the companies selling lasers or fillers or Botox or whatever they are using. Let's make the money. Something has to be done!

There is another aspect to all of this; and that is that there are procedures that are beginning to appear that are made for marketing, PR, and advertising but have no scientific basis or consistent scientific data to back them up. And there are a lot of them!

INFOMERCIAL AND DIRECTV

Well, they have to fill the airways with something. There once were three choices to watch on television (ABC, CBS, and NBC), and now with over five hundred channels, and most of them on twenty-four hours a day, there are hours and hours to fill. The infomercial industry is more than happy to fill that gap, and you can see any number of them especially during the night and on the weekends, but there is almost always one available at any time, and a great deal of them have to do with skin care and beauty. Why? Because this is a very visual form of a message. You can see the skin, and the message is easy to get across to the consumers. And it is very lucrative!

I have been in infomercials, have produced infomercials, and can give you a great deal of insight into this field that is made to inform and particularly sell. There are some very reputable companies in this field, and there are unscrupulous people here as there are in every field of endeavor, but this one is very enticing.

First of all, let's look at the infomercial itself. What is an infomercial? You would think it is a thirty-minute show on television that informs and tries to sell some type of product. Actually, an infomercial is three different sets of information separated by what is termed a "call to action"—an attempt to get you to buy something. The informative segment usually has an expert that may or may not have developed the skin-care product being discussed, and most certainly, a celebrity spokesperson. You must remember that the spokesperson is a celebrity and not an expert whose sole purpose is to keep you from using your remote control to switch channels and knows very little or nothing about the product and may not even have even used the product that is being sold. If you can identify with the celebrity, then things are that much better. I like her, so she must have good products, so I will buy it—that is one of the hooks of the infomercial. The most important characteristic of the celebrity spokesperson for the infomercial world is what is called "the Q factor." This number is made up of two parts: how recognizable is the person (how well known) and how well liked. So a company would not want to hire your next-door neighbor no matter how likable she is because she is not recognizable. On the other hand, an infomercial would never be done with OJ Simpson as the

MELVIN L. ELSON M. D.

spokesperson since he is very well known and recognizable but not well liked.

Another one is the testimonial. Women come on raving about the benefits they received, and most of them are sincere, but they received it for free and will continue to receive it for free which may skew their judgment a bit. Some of them, though, really have their lives changed, and I remember one woman in an infomercial that I was associated with who gained self-confidence, lost weight, and really changed her whole life because of a skin-care program that I developed and what the infomercial was selling. Was the program that good? Maybe, but the point is she believed it and believed in the spokesperson. Although the products were good and really did work, they did not need to be. She only needed to believe that they did, and this is a very important aspect to the infomercial and DirecTV business.

The biggest hook that the infomercial business has is that you are being offered a great deal, and it is guaranteed or even free! Well, let's look at this. The call to action usually states that you will be billed in a certain period of time for a certain amount of money for the product, but I have seen those that state that you only pay shipping and handling for a free trial and then bill you after what they call "the trial period." Honest? No. Allowed by the FTC? No. Is it done? Yes. Watch out for this, and when you call that toll free number even at two in the morning, be sure to ask when you are going to be billed and how much. There will also be the opportunity for you to buy more products just because you called—the so-called up sell. These add on to the cost of your purchase and may or may not be something you really want. But everything is guaranteed. That is true, but a great majority of dissatisfied customers simply don't fool with trying to get their money back. That is one of the most important aspects of not only infomercials but all of the other venues where there are guarantees, mail-in rebates, and all the other things that take action. Most people just don't fool with it, leaving the one who offered the rebate, guarantee, etc. with the money. And don't forget, you must call in the next fifteen minutes to get the special offer. Ever notice how many times you see the same infomercial over and over again with the same pitch, only fifteen minutes? There is the other ploy to get you to call and not procrastinate. Only the first one hundred callers will get free shipping and handling. Not so. All callers will be treated as if they are in the first one hundred and get free shipping and handling.

Don't get me wrong. Some of the products are actually very beneficial, and some have undergone extensive testing before getting on air to prove that they actually do what they say they are going to do and that they are safe. It is the manner in which it is presented that is often the problem.

Probably the most successful of all skin-care products in the infomercial world is Proactive, the acne treatment product. The reasons are simple. They chose a product for a very common condition—acne—and used known items that work—benzoyl peroxide and peroxide—chose attractive dermatologists to pitch and believable spokespersons, and voila, millions of dollars worth of product sold, now present even in machines in airports and in the inserts you get with your credit card. Great marketing and the product works in most cases. But can you get the same thing at the drugstore? Of course, you can; but you have to go to the drugstore, and you have to go back to get more and on and on and on. And there is a big difference between the local pharmacist telling you it works versus an attractive dermatologist or two and a well-known star.

If you are flipping through channels and happen to come across a celebrity hawking a skin-care line, just stop a second and think. Do I really want this and believe that it works, or am I just wishing it were true because of the celebrity? Realize that you do not need to hurry. No matter when you decide to order, you will be one of the first x number of callers to receive free shipping or whatever the first callers get. If you do call, you will be bombarded with the pitch for up sells, products linked to the main one that increase the sales and profits for the infomercial company. Ask them if they have a sample, and if not, then think about it. You can always order later. Remember, they will sign you up to receive product automatically every thirty to sixty days, whatever their gimmick is, and you do not have to do that either. Tell them you only want the first order, and then if you decide that you like the product, and it does what they said it would, and it is worth the money, if you want to sign up for automatic shipments, you can. The primary thing that they are trying to do is to make you hurry, make you think that if you do not sign up now and get everything and get it automatically, then you won't be able to in the future. Trust me, they will always be willing to take your money no matter when you call or under what circumstances.

DirecTV is another way of selling you product, and although you may think you are watching a live show, you may not really be. I have been involved with this also. Again, the products may be good, but it is the energy provided by the host or hostess and the deal you are getting that really is selling the product. There are so many of these direct selling TV channels now, and you can buy virtually anything on them; but as far as skin care is concerned, most of the products are not going to cause any harm, although for the most part, they are not going to make you as youthful and as beautiful as you think they are going to do. Some people actually become addicted to these types of sales programs and do not shop anywhere else. I know one woman who has one of the DirecTV channels on speed dial!

Then there is the issue of continuity. The first sale is just to get you in, but when you continue to get product month after month, that is when they really make money, so be sure that you only sign up for what you want. If you are getting a trial offer, make certain that you will not be sent more products in the future. If you want to sign up to get product on an ongoing basis, then by all means do so; but if you don't, don't get coerced into doing so.

THE MEDISPA

This is another new entity that has come alive in the last couple of decades. This area has become so large, so confusing, and so competitive that a dermatologist in New York even trademarked the term "Medispa," so many times, you will see medical spa or just medspa. It is amazing the turf battle that is occurring in this arena! Always protect your turf even if it is really not yours to protect.

There are so many of these so-called medical spas opening all over the country. Why is that? Because there are so many patients (customers) who desire cosmetic procedures and products that there is no way they can be seen by the few dermatologists and plastic surgeons in this country.

This type of business venture takes many forms. Some are merely extensions of dermatologists' offices or plastic surgeons or facial plastic surgeons. They are set up to provide services that are desired by patients but not provided in standard clinical settings—facials, body treatments, water treatments, massage, etc. These also serve as outlets to sell cosmetic and cosmeceutical products to the patients. Generally, these are the most legitimate and properly staffed venues with everything available in one location, sort of a one-stop shop. It has the advantage for the doctor to be able to control everything in your cosmetic care, from the skin-care products you are using to your filling material and Botox to the surgical procedures you may be having. *But* you must really be careful. Sure, it is convenient for you to be able to go to one location for everything, but there are places out there opened by doctors as an extension of their offices simply to increase their income without a great deal of concern for you. Know who is doing what to you. There are doctors, nurses, and aestheticians in these sites, but it is up to you to know who is doing what to you, and it is your right to know. It is your body, and things are being done to you. This type of medical spa in or part of a dermatologist's or plastic surgeon's office ought to be the most trustworthy and probably is, but you still have to be careful. Nurses should not be doing surgical procedures and aestheticians should not be injecting anything. Nowhere in the United States is it legal for an aesthetician to inject filling materials or Botox, but it is done. So ask! There are also plenty of free-standing sites that are not combined with physicians who are experts in the cosmetic field, and they are becoming more and more common. In some of the beachfront cities in California, I saw two or three so-called medispas every block. You can bet they are not all staffed by knowledgeable physicians, and some probably have never had any contact with any doctor of any sort.

There is such a big problem with malpractice costs in this country that many doctors are looking for sources of revenue away from high-risk areas. This is particularly true in states such as Florida and in specialties such as OB-GYN. Contributing to this problem is the shortage of dermatologists in certain areas of the country, and this has become a critical problem in Florida in particular. So a medical spa will open and be staffed by a doctor among others, but the doctor is not trained in the nuances of cosmetic procedures, cosmetic surgery, how to take care of the skin, and what to do in case something goes wrong. If pressed, they will say they have been trained by either a company or even in medical meetings to do certain procedures, but that is no substitute for years of training and expertise that the dermatologist brings to the table in all aspects of evaluating and treating aging skin, especially the aging face. In some states, laws are being passed that these medical spas may employ all kinds of personnel and doctors, but the medical director must be a dermatologist or plastic surgeon. So be sure there is a qualified, board-certified dermatologist or plastic surgeon in charge of the medical spa where you are and that everything that is being done is overseen by the aestheticians, nurses and doctors. Because of the popularity of cosmetic procedures, the increasing population of baby boomers, and the availability of new and advanced techniques, the so-called medspas are opening even if they do not have doctors of any type associated with them. The staff will tell you that they are trained in skin care, usually by the companies whose products they sell and that they are experts in filling materials, Botox, chemical peelings, etc. Nothing could be farther from the truth. You should not walk out of these places that do not have any doctors present and doing the procedures; you should run.

You must always remember that it is not only that you will waste your money in places like these, but even worse, if something significant goes wrong (infection, severe bruising, burns, etc.), they are not trained to take care of problems such as these. You may very well end up not only with a cosmetic procedure that did not help your appearance, you may actually look significantly worse!

So when you are considering going to a medispa or medspa or whatever they are called, make sure that the staff, which includes a physician, preferably with a medical director who is a dermatologist or plastic surgeon, is there and is going to at least oversee your care. Never choose to have any cosmetic procedure or work of any sort done simply because it is less expensive. In this area as well as most others, you get what you pay for.

After experiencing and researching the medical spa business, I have seen some very disturbing trends. At first, I thought that the major problem was going to be with aestheticians overstepping their boundaries and performing procedures that they should not and even nurses doing things that they should not be doing. However, for the most part, I have seen that these are basically very dedicated individuals who want to do what they have been trained to do and want to do an effective, safe job. There are two problems that I have seen come to the fore. The first is that someone or some entity owns this medspa. If it is associated with a dermatologist's office or a plastic surgeon, then you know who is in charge and what is basically going on. But more and more, these spas are popping up, owned by entrepreneurial adventurers whose main, and perhaps, only goal is to get patients (clients) in the door. The methods that are used are probably acceptable in many forms of business ventures but not in medicine, and this is something they simply do not understand and really do not want to. The other significant issue is somewhat of a surprise (at least to me). I have already mentioned the plethora of various medical specialties or nonspecialties lending doctors to these spas. What I did not expect is to see the change in some of these doctors (or is it really a change?). All of a sudden, they have become experts by being a medical director of a medical spa. No qualifications, very little training, and certainly no clue as to what to do in the event of a problem with a procedure, etc. I have even seen them claim to be plastic surgeons and present themselves as such. These are very dangerous individuals, and the only way to avoid such a situation is that if the medical director is not a board-certified dermatologist or plastic surgeon, just stay away. There are enough choices that you do not have to risk going to such a place regardless of the marketing they do and the discounts and all the other things that they offer to get you in the door.

In actuality, most Americans are pretty smart. In a survey conducted in 2006, most females surveyed thought that nonphysician-owned medical spas were not safe. 78 percent rated medical credentials as one of the most important aspects in considering whether or not to go to one of these. *But* they did not specify what kind of doctor should be there or the level of training that should be required. Actually, it is probably a great deal safer to have an experienced nurse or nurse practitioner under the direct supervision of a dermatologist or a plastic surgeon deal with your cosmetic issues than a physician from a noncore specialty who may or may not have any training.

Another red flag—the offer of discounts, coupons, or free services to get you in the door. They may also offer you a free service if you bring in your friends. All types of things are going on. Don't fall for it! These people act like they are selling used cars. Just stay away from them.

One thing you might be thinking is that, well, you can just go in and get something done for free and then not have to ever go back, but you could be harmed in that so-called free treatment. *Just stay away*!

Anytime you see another coupon in the mail for a discount on Botox or a chemical peel or anything else in one of these medispa locations, do the right thing. Throw it in the trash!

REALLY, HOW BAD COULD IT BE?

T he best way for me to let you know how bad things could be with a medical spa is for me to relate an absolutely true experience. A few years ago, I was approached by a group of investors who told me they were going to open and develop a chain of upscale medical spas that would have all the latest scientifically based medical procedures, staffed by qualified, trained medical personnel from the doctors to the nurses to the aestheticians and all the support staff, be the best at everything that was done, have the best equipment and all the latest developments from the world of cosmeceuticals. I was to train the doctors in the use of Botox, filling materials, how to evaluate the patient and the aging face, source skin-care products, and recommend what should and should not be done and what should be used. They had found what they said was a new type of face-lift that was minimally invasive, lasted as long as a conventional face-lift without the downtime or side effects, and results were comparable, developed by a physician (not a plastic or cosmetic surgeon) who had not presented the data at any scientific meeting and had not had his data published in any scientific journal, but they had seen the results and they were phenomenal.

I thought this was a wonderful idea, so I agreed and started treating patients there and obtaining skin-care products for them to sell and to oversee what was going on. Well, it did not take long to figure out what was going on. A doctor who had no experience in cosmetic or plastic surgery but was trained by the inventor of the procedure was hired to perform this new procedure. After a number of months and after I had observed what was going on, I came to the following conclusions: The doctor did not know what she was doing, and the procedure did not even work. I demanded a meeting of the board and was astounded to find out that the board consisted of lawyers, accountants, businessmen, and entrepreneurs, not one medical person of any sort! I told them that they were harming people and should do something immediately. Of course, they did not believe me but did have a review of all the charts and found at least a 40 percent side-effect rate, some of which were severe and that most of the patients had the "magic procedure" redone because it did not provide the benefits that they were marketing and advertising. They stopped the procedure, fired the doctor who was doing the surgery, but remained in business, doing some minor procedures with other personnel. As of this writing, they have not closed their doors but are contemplating in closing up the shop. One of the things that you can depend on is that over time, whatever the locale and whatever the situation, a reputation is earned.

SO WHAT CAN YOU DO?

here is so much distortion of the market and so many pitfalls
that it seems impossible to be able to trust anyone or anything
in the beauty industry. But you do want to look and feel your
best. So there must be some guidelines that can be followed so you do
not have to simply throw in the towel and age gracefully.

First and foremost, use common sense. If you or your family are
already in the hands of a reputable dermatologist or plastic surgeon,
seeks his or her advice or expertise in what you want to accomplish.
Almost all dermatologists or plastic surgeons in the United States are
already providing the services that you are seeking or the evaluation
that you might need. If you do not have one of these doctors in your
armamentarium already, seek one out and remember to get referrals
from your family and friends, not necessarily from your personal
physician unless you have ways of checking out the doctor to whom
you have been referred, and certainly not from the yellow pages or from
advertisements. But not everyone in this country has easy access to one
of these doctors. That is where the conundrum comes in. What do you
do? There are a number of avenues you could go down. If you simply
cannot get to one of these core physicians, then you have the choice of
trying another specialty or the medical spa. If you are thinking of going
to a doctor out of the core specialties of dermatology, plastic surgery, or
facial or ophthalmic plastic surgery, see if that doctor does have some
specialized training from the American Academy of Cosmetic Surgery
or the American Academy of Aesthetic Medicine. Even though these
are not boards that are recognized by the American Board of Medical
Specialties, at least you would have some indication that there is some
minimum level of expertise in the basic cosmetic procedures such as
Botox injections, fillers, some laser, and other noninvasive procedures.
But how do you know how experienced he really is? Ask, ask, ask.
Ask him. Ask any friends or relatives you know who may have seen
him, and then decide whether you want to be seen by him and for a
procedure.

If the doctor is already your primary care physician, and you are
thinking about letting that doctor become your cosmetic physician
and/or surgeon, then check him/ her out as if he/she is a brand new

doctor. Do not be intimidated, and the doctor should want to tell you all about the qualifications that are there for the things that you are seeking. If your gynecologist is a wonderful doctor but has taken no extra courses and no steps to become qualified in the world of cosmetic procedures, go elsewhere. But where?

Here comes the medical spa. As you will remember, there are medical spas in all types of situations and venues. If one is associated with a dermatologist or plastic surgeon, and the doctor performs the procedure or is on the premises when his nurse does, and you can check out the facility as to what kind of results they get, then go for it. If there is no doctor there and if aestheticians are doing medical procedures such as injections and chemical peels, don't go there. If the primary doctor in charge of any facility calling themselves a medical spa is not a dermatologist, plastic surgeon, or facial plastic surgeon and is available, simply stay away. A gynecologist or an emergency room doctor in charge of a medical spa is simply not going have the expertise to treat you, and you are certainly asking for trouble in the event that something does go wrong.

True, there are some who have been trained by other physicians in courses and preceptorships, and they may be qualified, so check them out. Ask where they have received the extra training to perform the procedures that you desire, and that allows them now to change from their previous specialty to the world of cosmetic surgery and medicine. Too often they just want to escape the insurance companies' low reimbursement and the outrageous fees for malpractice insurance. That may be good enough for them, but it is not good enough for you. Ask, ask, and ask again.

THE CALIFORNIA INQUISITION

To point out some of the real problems in this area (all of the cosmetic world), let me give you a real example that occurred just recently. I am involved in teaching botulinum toxin (Botox) and filling materials for one of the societies that attempts to give some expertise to doctors who are adding cosmetic procedures to their practices or even going into cosmetic surgery and medicine completely.

There was a meeting scheduled in California that was supposed to last for three days with me teaching Botox and fillers, someone teaching how to use lasers and someone teaching chemical peels. When I got to the hotel, I was told that there were two people from the California board of medical examiners wanting to meet with me. I met with them, and we discussed what was going on. I am licensed to practice medicine in five states and one foreign country and the president of the society is licensed in Europe. Since my license was not in California, I was told that I could lecture but not inject a patient or demonstrate at all. I agreed to do that, and to make a long story short, we just cancelled the conference. Here we were with doctors who actually wanted to learn how to do things properly at least at a minimum, but these people from California were not interested in that.

I told them about all the problems with people doing procedures who have no training at all, many of whom were not any type of doctor, and I was told that was not their area. Think about it. Here, we have two agents from California not really caring about whether or not people are trained at all in working in the so-called medispas, most of which are a problem in California. They were much more interested in talking with one of the world's experts on cosmetic procedures (me—and they admitted that) about not having a piece of paper from California.

During our conversation, they made a number of ludicrous statements indicating that they did not even know what they were talking about:

Botox is a drug—no it is not; it is a biologic toxin.

Juvéderm is a dangerous material—it is safe and FDA approved and used all around the world with no problem.

Medical materials cannot be shipped across state lines—if that were true Botox could only be used in California where it is manufactured.

I (since I have no CA license) cannot even touch a needle in California—this is false too.

And it goes on and on. They simply want $2,000 for a CA license, and that is the name of the game. People doing things such as aestheticians injecting in medispas or a woman with no training of any sort injecting silicone from an auto repair shop—they just can't fool with those sorts of things.

This is the type of ridiculous behavior that is going on and one of the reasons you must be very careful when choosing someone to treat your aging skin.

MEDICAL TOURISM

One of the interesting consequences of globalization is the development of an entirely new industry—medical tourism. Although this began with traveling to Asia to obtain hip replacement, heart bypass surgery, or other major medical/ surgery issues, this has translated into patients seeking out cosmetic procedures in far corners of the globe. Why is this being done? There are many reasons. Certainly, one is cost. Many Americans are having some difficult times at the moment, and health care should not suffer, whether it is so-called necessary health care or cosmetic services. Two of the most common areas that are close, easy to get to, and provide excellent medical care are some venues in Mexico and Costa Rica. Long known for its beautiful scenery, eco-friendly atmosphere, and excellent delivery of medical care, a new era is dawning in Costa Rica. A US-based company, Appearance International, is establishing a cosmetic surgery clinic in Costa Rica to provide not only the best medical care possible for dermatologic cosmetic procedures and products as well as plastic surgery but also provides an oversight never before available in this arena. The company has established a concierge system whereby once a patient makes the initial contact, the concierge handles all the arrangements for the patient to undergo a full consultation with a certified plastic surgeon and dermatologist in the clinic to determine what is best for the patient. Additionally, all aspects of travel, etc. are arranged not only for the patient but also any family members or accompanying individuals so that they can not only share the experience with the patient but also schedule vacation time and any activities they desire. As opposed to other service companies such as travel agents, the concierge service then follows the patient through the procedure and aftercare on site. Upon returning to the United States, follow up continues, and that concierge remains available to the patient at any time thereafter related to that particular visit or arranging others or any questions regarding medical care. This is the first time there is continuity of medical care in the medical tourism industry.

The company was founded by three individuals. It is the brain child of Terry Knapp, MD, a world renowned plastic surgeon who founded Collagen Corporation, has established a number of successful companies over the years and performs a great deal of charity work throughout the world especially in third world countries. Torrie Sullivan is a holder of a master's degree in medical tourism and brings the expertise needed and the contacts to guarantee that the highest quality service is in place from either upscale hotels or the best hospitals in the area. I am the third individual involved in establishing this company. We do not only oversee the local physicians who are dermatologists and plastic surgeons as opposed to nonskilled physicians, but we are also committed to providing the best service, the safest proven cosmetic procedures, and the most advance skin care products that are hypoallergenic, scientifically proven, and packaged in an eco-friendly manner. The company is also committed to be a green company in all venues and will provide a portion of the profits to be used in the local community for medical care of the underprivileged.

In addition to Costa Rica, clinics with the same characteristics will be formed in Mexico, Singapore, and Dubai. Further clinics and developments will unfold as these first become operational. Although medical tourism has been present and flourishing in many venues over the last couple of decades up until this point, up until recently the decision regarding medical tourism has been a hit and miss situation with the admonition always present of "buyer beware." There is no doubt that the United States has one of the best, if not the best, medical care available anywhere in the world. However, the system is broken and remains so. So much of our population cannot afford the myriad of services available. That is why joint replacements and even heart bypass surgery has become so prevalent at one of the major hospitals in Bangkok. This venue is staffed by well-trained doctors, and the hospital looks more like a resort than a hospital. It is beautiful, and the medical care is safe, effective, and at a cost of a fraction of the same procedure performed in the United States. But what about cosmetic procedures?

Just as patients from the United States are going to clinics all over the world for hip replacements and heart bypass surgery, so are they also going for all types of cosmetic procedures, from face-lifts to eye jobs to breast implants and tummy tucks. And patients are coming to the United States as well. There are many reasons that this business is literally booming all over the world. Some are going to seek a procedure at a lower cost. Some are able to combine the surgical procedure with a recuperative vacation and perhaps save a little money or maybe no, but the point may be to have a vacation, enjoy, and return home and certainly look rested as never before. But in the world of cosmetic surgery and aesthetic medicine, there is always lurking caveat emptor. Buyer, beware. Studies performed by the American Academy of Plastic Surgeons has shown that a side-effect rate of up to 20 percent is not at all unusual. Now you really have to be careful choosing not just the location for a vacation or a blissful rest but also a surgeon and a facility from perhaps halfway across the world!

There are many websites and organizations and travel agencies at your disposal, and more are appearing virtually every day. One of the ways to possibly circumvent problems is referral by your physician in your home country—US or otherwise, and even better, a friend or family member who can recommend someone and his facility from personal experience. This is not always possible and societies such as the American Academy of Plastic Surgeons and the American Academy of Dermatology are hesitant to recommend doctors outside the US. But now there has developed a way that you can avail yourself of the best information that is out there regarding aesthetic medicine and surgery—Appearance International. Based in the United States, this is the first entity to establish a global group medical practice in the field of aesthetic medicine and surgery. The physicians forming this group practice are all board certified in their specialty, and everyone is certified in a core specialty—dermatology, plastic surgery, or facial plastic surgery—no obstetricians or emergency room doctors looking for a new life. These doctors are all not only qualified, they are highly qualified and among the best in their respective fields and practice in facilities that meet the standards set by both Appearance International and all the appropriate governmental and regulatory authorities. Appearance International offers a number of unique services. When first contacted by a patient, a personal concierge is assigned to that patient to take care of all the needs from travel arrangements to appointment with appropriate physicians at the proper facilities to making any and all arrangements for travel, lodging, and even sightseeing for you and your family and will follow you all the way through the procedure and beyond to be certain that you achieve the safest and best medical care available anywhere in the world. And there is always the remote possibility that there will be a side effect from the procedure. In that event, the company will be certain you get the best care to alleviate the problem. Either with the out-of-country physician or your home physician, you will be taken care of, and the cost will be covered by Appearance International.

BOARD CERTIFICATION

This issue has come up a number of times in this book and is an important issue that plays a significant role in your choice of a physician not only for your cosmetic needs but also for all your medical issues. Basically, board certification was set up decades ago to be certain that doctors who trained in a particular specialty actually developed the skills and knowledge to practice that specialty.

To become board eligible (this is a term you will see when a physician has not yet completed the examinations and become certified), a physician must complete a specified program of training after medical school. The training varies with individual specialties, e.g., dermatology requires a year's internship and three years of residency to become board eligible. Then one applies to take the board exam, which is an intense written and oral examination. If one does not pass the examination, he can remain board eligible for a period of time (varies with the specialty), but if the doctor takes the exam and fails it again, he cannot remain board eligible and must get more training. Once all requirements are met and the examinations are passed, then that doctor is board certified.

However, as in many things having to do with certification and qualifications in medicine, things are not really that simple. The board certification process has been ongoing for decades and the *true* boards are under the auspices of the American Board of Medical Specialties of which there are twenty-four recognized boards. This is important to understand because there are so-called boards that have been established outside the control of this organization and do not meet the same standards set by the American Board of Medical Specialties. Although some doctors may take courses and learn some basics of a new field of endeavor, there are gaps in knowledge that are important to taking care of patients. When a physician is certified in his specialty, that is the only board certification there is, and he may study other disciplines and become minimally proficient, but he remains board certified in his original specialty. For example, someone who is board certified in OB-GYN (completed all the training and passed written and oral examination in that specialty) may take courses in cosmetic procedures and attend conferences emphasizing cosmetic procedures, but he is board certified only in OB-GYN. There is no such recognized board as cosmetic surgery. So if he decides to change the emphasis of his practice for one reason or another, then that does not change his qualifications. You must be careful when you see advertisements for services offered by board-certified cosmetic surgeons or see ads for cosmetic surgery stating that the doctor in control of the facility is board certified. The question you should ask is in which specialty are they board certified in.

Unfortunately, you cannot always determine whether the doctor who is presenting the credentials is certified in a specialty that is approved by the American Board of Medical Specialties and that the training he received meets the *minimal* standards set by the medical community. Physicians who are certified by the American Board of Cosmetic Surgery and the American Academy of Aesthetic Medicine may have some training, but their certification is not recognized by the medical community. If you are seeking a cosmetic consultation or procedure, you should be certain that the doctor is board certified in one of the following: plastic surgery, dermatology, ophthalmology, or ear, nose, and throat (facial plastic surgery). Any other designation, whether of a specialty you recognize or an organization that may not sound right to you, should raise your suspicion.

QUESTIONS TO ASK YOUR DERMATOLOGIST

Are you board certified in dermatology?
How many of these procedures have you performed?
What are the side effects?
How much is it going to cost?
Who is going to perform the procedure: you or your assistant?
How do I get in touch with you if I have a side effect?
Where did you train?
Have you taught this procedure at a meeting or published it in a
  journal?

QUESTIONS TO ASK YOUR PLASTIC SURGEON

Are you board certified in plastic surgery?
Where is this procedure going to be performed?
What type of anesthesia will you use?
Who will administer the anesthesia?

Is the operating room located in your office or the hospital?
Is the operating room Medicare approved?
When will you see me back?
How do I get in touch with you directly if I need to?

THINGS YOU MUST TELL YOUR DOCTOR

Medications you are on including over-the-counter medicines
Vitamins, supplements, herbs, etc. that you take
Past surgeries
Any illness in the past that require hospitalization
Any allergies to anything, not just medications
Why you want this procedure done
Complications you have had in the past procedures
Have you arranged aftercare, if necessary

QUESTIONS FOR THE MEDSPA

Who owns the spa?
What type of doctor is the medical director?
If not a core physician, why not?
If not, what is his field of specialty?
If a core physician, is he board certified?
Is there an operating room that is sterile?
What types of anesthesia do you use here?
What types of procedures do your aestheticians perform?
What if I have a side effect from something done here?
How do you handle after hour calls?

QUESTIONS TO ASK AT THE COSMETIC COUNTER

How long have you been selling skin-care products?
How were you trained to do this?
What are the key ingredients in—?
Is there any animal testing done on your products?
Is this fragrance free or perfume free?
What if I have a reaction to this?
Is it dermatologist tested and dermatologist recommended?
What is the shelf life of this product?

Were clinical trials performed on this product?
If I don't like it, can I get my money back?

WHAT TO ASK ABOUT THE PRODUCT

Is it FDA approved?
What is it made of?
Is the syringe fresh (used on no one else)?

WHAT DO THEY REALLY MEAN?

There are many ways to use words that convey things that we believe they are saying; when in actuality, the meaning is quite different. This is very common in the labeling and in the marketing and advertising of cosmetic and cosmeceuticals products. This chapter will present what something says, what we think it means, and what it actually means.

What it says: Prevents the signs of aging

What it means: Contains sunscreen

What it says: Dermatologist approved

What it means: Dermatologist is a consultant.

What it says: All natural

What it means: Active ingredients are derived from natural sources; may contain artificial or chemical fragrance, color or preservatives.

What it says: Fragrance free

What it means: No detectable scent but may contain fragrance to mask other smells in the product.

What it says: Data on file

What it means: Tests done and information internal to the company; may or may not be from a reputable source and may not really support what the company is saying in their advertising.

What it says: Contains antioxidants

What it means: Contains vitamin C or similar agents but may or may not be effective.

What it says: No animal testing

What it means: Exactly what it says.

What it says: Moisturizing

What it means: Contains water

What it says: Organic

What it means: Active ingredients and most excipients are derived from organic products—natural, environmentally safe.

What it says: Contains vitamin E

What it means: Does contain it but usually not enough to matter in the formulation.

What it says: As seen on TV
What it means: Simply that the product has been marketed on TV; means nothing.
What it says: pH balanced
What it means: Amount of acidity adjusted to be the same as the skin, slightly acid, so it has less tendency to dry the skin.
What it says: Does not contain PABA
What it means: Labeling on a sunscreen says that it does not contain this chemical as it was used in sunscreens in the past, and there were allergies.
What it says: Sunscreen is waterproof.
What it means: Some resistance to washing off. No sunscreen is waterproof.

DR E.'S QUICK GUIDE

BEAUTY, HEALTH, AND WELL-BEING FOR LIFE

Every morning, apply a sunscreen with an A and B block and SPF15–30.

Never smoke cigarettes.

Drink moderately—one or two glasses of wine every evening.

Do not take sleeping pills even over-the-counter ones.

There is only one moisturizer for the skin—water.

The sun puts out two types of UV light that get to earth: B, which causes skin cancer and sunburn, and A, which causes melanoma and aging.

Tanning beds put out only UVA, so they say they are safe. Really?

UVA also causes cataracts. Always wear sunglasses that specifically block UVA. More expensive but worth it.

Best eye makeup and mascara remover? Johnson's baby shampoo (straight).

Best way to moisturize your face: At night, apply a little water and cover with a thin film of Vaseline. In the morning, it will be smooth as can be.

Take one baby aspirin every day.

For men one without iron, take a multivitamin every day.

Get outside every day for fifteen minutes even if you do nothing out there.

Get thirty minutes vigorous exercise at least three times a week outside if at all possible.

Vigorous exercise means you can talk during activity, but it's not easy.

Eat breakfast. No time? *Eat breakfast.*

Do not use soap on your face. Use a beauty bar or cleanser. There is a difference!

Do not use antibacterial wipes in your home. They may produce super germs.

Want to create a new habit? Do it for five weeks without failing.

Drink at least 32 oz of water a day. Water, not just liquids.

Weigh every day, gain a pound, *lose* it!

Know the seven danger signs of cancer.

Testing makeup on your hands makes no sense unless you are going to wear makeup on your hands.

Talk to God. He is listening.

Use your vacation time.

Apply retinol after shaving legs or face to prevent razor bumps.

The worst place to find a doctor? The yellow pages.

The worst place for medical information? The Internet.

Be sure the doctor that you have chosen is board certified in the specialty in which he is performing the procedure. You don't want a gynecologist injecting your Botox any more than you want your dermatologist delivering your baby.

The best place to find a doctor? From one of his patients and not another doctor.

A doctor's reputation is earned, and he deserves what he has earned one way or the other.

The worst way to choose a doctor? Price.

Insurance companies are not there to help you. They are there to make money.

The SPF in moisturizers and even makeup is not enough for adequate sun protection.

Botox should not be injected into lines but into muscles that cause the lines.

If Botox injections are painful, they are done incorrectly.

Botox is currently approved in the US only for frown line treatment.

Hyaluronic acid injections for lines and wrinkles (like Restylane) are far superior to collagen injections.

Retin-A is vitamin A acid and was invented because topical vitamin A could not be stabilized in the 1960s.

Retinol is vitamin A and can now be stabilized, but not all products contain stable retinol.

If a vitamin C product turns brown, it is no longer effective regardless of what the manufacturer says.

Vitamin E has no effect on scars. Might as well rub motor oil on the scar or area of surgery.

The definition of an aesthetician will vary from state to state.

The purpose of a chemical peel is to burn the skin and allow it to heal back smoother and more even.

Acids are used to perform chemical peels. The stronger the acid, the deeper the peel, the better the results, but the more likely there are to be side effects.

A lot of doctors receive training in how to use a laser over a weekend course. Check out his experience.

Three best things to do for your face: Use sunscreen every morning, use retinol every night, and don't smoke.

Nothing you can put on hair or nails makes them healthier. They are both products of the skin and are not alive.

Peptides are nothing but pieces of protein, and no data has proven if they are effective when applied to the skin.

Silicone injections are not safe, and side effects may be delayed for decades.

With new fillers for wrinkles, there is no longer any reason to have collagen from cows injected.

Topical vitamin K can prevent bruises and make them go away faster.

Triple antibiotic ointments are one of the most common causes of allergy.

The vast majority of the cost in most prestige cosmetics is in the packaging and marketing, not the actual product.

Retin-A has been shown to be effective in the treatment of stretch marks.

Electrolysis will not make hair grow back coarser.

Newer techniques in hair transplantation look totally natural.

Minoxidil does work to regrow hair and prevent hair loss especially in women.

Applying retinol to the skin before using any product in the area makes it work better.

Avoid Botox parties. This is a medical procedure.

Products with glycolic acid help smooth the skin a little but also help other products get in better.

The glue used to apply artificial nails destroys the natural nail.

The perfect female face brings out only the eyes and the lips.

A face-lift is done because the picture has slipped out of the frame.

A mini face-lift is like a mini pregnancy!

Sculptra injections are said to be permanent. Not true.

Sleep lines occur from putting the face into the pillow in the same position every night.

A simple way to improve lines that are not too deep is to apply a piece of tape over the line each night before bed.

Sun damage accounts for about 80 percent of what we call the aging face.

There is no real evidence that antiperspirants are related to breast cancer.

Antiperspirants stop sweating whereas deodorants simply mask odor.

Acne and other complexion problems have many causes; chocolate is not one of them.

There are no products that can be applied to the skin that work like Botox.

A face-lift cannot be delayed with injections of any type.

Intrinsic aging (skin wearing out) doesn't begin to occur until the seventh decade of life.

Almost all signs of aging are extrinsic and can be prevented.

To prevent bruising from cosmetic procedures, apply vitamin K cream twice daily for a week prior to the procedure.

To prevent new blood vessels from forming after leg vein treatment, apply vitamin K cream after bathing.

Learn how to do self breast examinations, and do them every day.

Aging hands are a giveaway that you have had procedures on the face.

Have a physical every year—a complete one.

Men should donate blood as often as possible. It decreases the chance of heart attacks.

Subscribe to the Mayo Clinic Health Letter.

The experts chosen for most local TV shows are paid advertisers.

Celebrity spokespeople are just that—celebrities, not experts.

Just because something is natural doesn't mean it is good for you.

Infomercials can guarantee products because they know that if they do not deliver, most people do not fool with a refund.

Labeling in the cosmetic industry is a game. A cosmetic product can state that it decreases the appearance of wrinkles but cannot say it decreases wrinkles.

As gravity affects the face, even the ears get longer.

With true aging, even the skull begins to get smaller.

Female pattern baldness or hair loss is actually more common than male.

If an optometrist or ophthalmologist can demonstrate that your visual fields are decreased due to overhanging skin, insurance will often pay for an eye job.

The more natural you look after a procedure the better.

After a face-lift, the face should be more round, not pulled tight.

As gravity affects our lips, the upper lip looks like it has disappeared. Where is it? Turned into the mouth.

If your doctor has an operating room in his office, ask if it is certified by Medicare even if you don't have Medicare.

If a doctor offers to help you cheat your insurance company by listing a cosmetic procedure as something else, simple—walk out!

Never allow someone in a hotel room from outside the US to inject anything into your face.

Cosmeceuticals are skin care products obtained without a prescription that do have benefits for the skin.

The FDA does not recognize the term "cosmeceuticals," but that does not mean it does not exist.

Nutraceuticals are substances taken by mouth and obtained without a prescription that have some benefit helping to remain healthy and youthful.

Data on file is a common term in the cosmetic industry and means that they have performed studies to support claims but have not made specific claims nor published the data.

The prescription Renova* is an emollient form of Retin-A*.

Renova is marketed for wrinkles and Retin-A for acne; otherwise, the active ingredient is the same.

When looking at ingredient lists of cosmetic products, remember that they start with the highest concentration and go to the lowest.

A vitamin is a substance necessary to maintain the body's health, but the body does not have the ability to manufacture and must get from an outside source.

God made skin to keep things out, and it does a very good job. The trick is to figure out how to get things applied to the skin make it work.

Microdermabrasion works as well as a rough washcloth—the emperor's new clothes!

On long-haul airline flights, spray your face with saline mist every hour or so.

After menopause, a woman will lose 30 percent of the collagen in her skin over time.

Collagen provides the framework that holds up the skin, like an erector set.

Elastic fibers allow the skin to move and it will snap back into place when the skin is young.

Hyaluronic acid is the best water holder in our skin, our eyes, and our joints or in cosmetic moisturizers.

Growth factors are very important in the skin but may be totally worthless in skin-care preparations.

Before buying anything from an infomercial or DirecTV, ask exactly what and when they are going to charge your credit card.

Continuity sales are where infomercials make their money. Only sign up for it if you really want it.

Glycolic acid is found in sugar cane, but the glycolic acid in almost all skin care products is chemically produced and is not natural.

Cleopatra bathed in milk to soften her skin, utilizing the skin softening benefits of lactic acid.

To soften dry cracked heels, moisten the area, apply Vaseline, and put on socks overnight.

Never have a cosmetic procedure for someone else, only for yourself.

Most common complaint from women wanting a cosmetic procedure: I am beginning to look like my mother.

Do not even think of cosmetic surgery during a very emotional period such as after the death of a loved one, a divorce, etc.

If you find a very comfortable pillow in a hotel, find out how you can order one.

Depression is not something you snap out of. If you are depressed, seek help

Practice safe sex 100 percent of the time.

Don't try and see the color of a foundation, eye shadow, etc. on your hand unless that is where you are going to use it.

To determine the true color of something you are buying at the cosmetic counter, go outside in the real light. Department store lights cast a blue color.

Enzyme peels derived from fruit and used in spas do help remove very superficial layers of the skin.

Papaya produces an enzyme called "papain," which can be used as an enzyme peel.

Pineapple produces an enzyme called "bromelain," which can be used as an enzyme peel.

Most doctors' offices that have their own private label products are simply cheap bulk products with the doctor's label.

Read labels just as carefully on cosmetics as you do on drugs, and follow the directions to the fullest.

Liposuction is not a treatment for obesity.

Just because an expert recommends something in a book or on TV does not mean it is right for you.

A doctor who never has a complication is a liar.

The most important characteristic of a good doctor is that he will take care of you if something goes wrong.

Everyone knows better-looking people get better tables at restaurants, but they also get better medical care.

The most important factor in determining your health and how long you will live is self-esteem.

Alternative medicine is beginning to be studied in major medical centers, but that is not an endorsement.

A study at Duke University showed that patients who were prayed for did better than those who were not.

Retin-A does not work by irritation. That is an unnecessary side effect.

Be careful of taking herbs, vitamins, or supplements. They may interact with medicine you are on.

Lapband surgery for weight loss has been proven effective and is much safer than stomach stapling or bypass.

Attend a skin cancer screening once a year even if your doctor checks you for skin cancer.

Know how to perform CPR on both adults and children.

If a mole changes in *any* way, see a dermatologist.

Plastic surgeons are not skin care experts.

Oprah is an expert—in promotion.

FDA approval does not necessarily mean there can be no problems from the approved item. Approval is based on data from a limited number of patients.

Although more expensive, organically grown fruits and vegetables are not necessarily more healthy.

In a blind taste test of water, including many bottled and city waters, New York City water came out on top.

Laughing is good for the way you feel, and it is good for your heart.

Vanilla-based perfume may cause pigment problems on exposure to the sun. Apply it to areas not exposed to the sun.

Use unscented laundry detergent and fabric softener.

Want to keep your blood pressure down? Pet a dog or a cat.

Injectable filling materials like collagen or Restylane can make lips more visible—like internal lip liner.

A combination of topical vitamin K and retinol has been shown to decrease the appearance of dark circles.

Stretch marks are actually little scars in the skin, not areas where the skin has stretched more than it can snap back.

Know how to perform the Heimlich maneuver.

Substituting pipe smoking or chewing tobacco for cigarettes substitutes mouth cancer for lung cancer.

Rosacea is not a sign of aging but a form of acne with a great deal of redness.

Anything that increases blood flow to the face (alcohol, emotions, etc.) will make rosacea worse.

Cellulite and obesity are not the same thing.

80 percent of women over eighteen have cellulite at one time or another during their lifetime.

Diet and exercise have no effect on the appearance of cellulite.

Studies that have shown low-fat diets have no effect on prevention of heart disease or cancer were poorly designed.

Apply bath oil to moist skin after a shower, and then pat dry to moisturize the skin.

You cannot ingest enough vitamins by mouth to get a high concentration for action in the skin.

A new filling material for wrinkles that is almost permanent, i.e., long lasting, has been approved by the FDA—Radiesse˚.

As the face ages, the bite changes, and cosmetic dentistry should be a factor in treating the aging face.

The sunken appearance of aging hands can be treated with fat injections or other injectables.

Chemical peels performed on the neck and chest have a much greater chance of side effects than the same peel done on the face.

A Swedish study claims that eating cultured yogurt decreases the chance of catching a cold.

A study at Duke University found that the magic number to keep fat from your midriff is eleven hours of exercise per week.

If you are under a lot of stress, you produce cortisol which will keep you from losing weight.

If you do not want to drink any alcohol, you can get antioxidants from grape juice or fresh grapes, especially black grapes.

The main difference between most of the skin-care products for women and those for men: packaging and marketing.

Three things that will make the most difference in your skin: Use a sunscreen every morning, apply retinol every night, and don't smoke.

Benzoyl peroxide remains one of the best treatments for acne.

ProActiv does work for acne most of the time.

There is no such thing as the best makeup. It is really all trial and error to find what is right for you.

Always wash your hands after applying retinol or an acid to your face prior to going to bed.

The best place for a man to shave is in the shower. The heat and moisture make for a closer, smoother, and safer shave.

If possible, avoid products containing sweet fragrances that remain on the skin as in shaving cream or moisturizers as these do attract insects.

The old adage about poison ivy is simple and is true—leaves of 3, let them be.

To relieve the pain from sunburn, apply compresses of ice cold milk.

You cannot change the lack of self-esteem you may have due to your upbringing, but don't pass it on.

Compliment at least one person every day.

Whenever a child comes to your door selling something—buy it.

Do not wear the same running shoes every day. Rotate.

Always run on the side facing the traffic so you can see the cars, and they can see you.

If you are running in the heat of the day in the summer, the white line is a little cooler than the asphalt.

If you have a choice between running on concrete or on asphalt, choose asphalt. It gives; concrete does not.

Onion extract (sold as Mederma) actually does improve the appearance of scars.

Asian and African-American skin respond differently to treatments for aging than Caucasian skin.

Age sixty is the new middle age, and eighty-five is the beginning of old age.

The most common cosmetic procedure now performed in the world is Botox injections.

Onion extract cream (Mederma) also improves the appearance of stretch marks.

Many times, a breast lift will provide better cosmetic results than breast implants.

Silicone breast implants have still not been approved for use by the FDA.

Saline breast implants are approved for breast augmentation but do not feel natural.

There is no link between hair dye and cancer.

There is no way to get rid of pores on the face.

The only way to shrink pores and to keep them as small as possible is to keep them clean and emptied out with a masque or a good facial.

The person who can spend the most time with you and help you the most with your skin is a knowledgeable aesthetician.

Once you find an esthetician who knows your skin and is taking good care of you, do not go seek another one.

Never have your skin care needs evaluated by someone behind a counter in a department store.

Some of the large cosmetic companies have very large and very good research departments producing good science.

There is no such thing as surgery without a scar.

Microdermabrasion is the emperor's new clothes of skin care.

There are prescription creams that can remove precancers and early cancer of the skin.

There is prevention for colon cancer. It is called colonoscopy.

Colonoscopy is not a painful procedure. The worst part is getting ready for it.

Keep a bag of walnuts around and reach for a handful every now and then—one of the healthiest things you can do.

Best antioxidant and cancer-fighting fruit—blueberries.

Do not trust blood pressure machines in stores to be completely accurate.

Free seminars given by doctors in the evening are more for marketing themselves and procedures than informational and educational.

Do not ever get a tattoo.

There is no way to completely remove a tattoo and leave no scar.

Make sure your dermatologist does a complete skin exam to check for skin cancer once a year. Have your birthday suit checked on your birthday.

If you can find a doctor who teaches a procedure to other doctors, he is the one you want to do that procedure on you.

The most difficult cosmetic problem to treat is uneven color of the skin.

If your insurance company turns down a claim you and your doctor believe they should pay, fight them. They often give in eventually.

Men should check themselves for testicular cancer in the shower. Find a lump; have it checked!

The worst reason not to go to the doctor: I was afraid that what I had was serious.

If you think you might be having a heart attack, chew an aspirin immediately. If you are OK, you wasted one aspirin. If you are not, it could save your life.

Check with an ophthalmologist about using a lubricating eye drop during long flights instead of saline drops.

Cosmetic dentistry is very important in reversing the signs of the aging face.

To avoid overeating and overspending in airports, take some fruit with you.

Men should see a urologist once a year for a checkup and PSA if over fifty.

Women do need to have pap smears every year.

Massage is one of the best ways to relax and increase circulation.

If you injure a joint or muscle, ice it for the first two days and apply moist heat after that.

An easy way to have ice to apply to an injury is to keep a small paper cup filled with water in the freezer. You can apply it without having to touch the ice.

Moist heat (like a specially made heating pad) penetrates deeper than dry heat.

To dry up blisters, apply compresses of a solution made of two tablespoons of white vinegar to a pint of water.

Avocados are full of fat—the good kind.

Eat fish, preferably cold water fish, at least twice a week.

When running in the windy cold weather, run into the wind if you can, and then when you turn around, the wind will be at your back while you are sweaty.

If you can afford one, a personal trainer is a good way to at least get you started on a good program of exercise.

A lot of people just don't know how and what to eat—if that is you see a registered dietician and find out. Check your local hospital.

To keep nipples from rubbing against clothing when running, apply Vaseline before you run. Also works if your thighs are rubbing together,

There is absolutely nothing approved for use during pregnancy. No procedure, no drug, no cosmeceutical, and no cosmetic.

Retinol (vitamin A) combined with topical vitamin K can improve dark spots on the skin and even out the color.

The reason acids are used in chemical peels and in skin-care products as opposed to alkali, which would also change the pH of the skin and peel it, is that alkali are not controllable.

The more colors of food on your plate, the healthier the food.

When in a foreign country, try to eat something you have never tried before. You might like it, but be sure that you know what it is.

Melatonin is probably ineffective in helping jet lag.

Try to get seven to eight hours sleep every night. Most Americans get only six, and the extra makes everything during the day more productive.

Exercise your brain using crossword puzzles or sudoku. Learn a foreign language.

Married men live longer than single men especially if they are happily married.

If you think you are old, you are, even if you are forty.

If you think you are young, you are, even if you are eighty.

It takes 3,500 calories to gain or lose a pound.

The more you move, the more calories you burn. Stand while on the phone, walk up steps, etc.

You use about one hundred calories moving through a mile—walking or running, fast or slow.

When traveling, the best exercise is swimming—not much to pack, no stress, good caloric use, and relaxing.

A good way to exercise and learn about a new city is to walk. Be sure where you are walking is safe.

If you want to look like a local instead of a tourist, buy a local language newspaper, and carry it under your arm.

To keep valuables safe in your hotel room, use the safe, leave the TV on, and put up the Do Not Disturb sign when you go out.

Walking actually helps minor arthritis pains. The movement and lubrication are important.

Keep two teaspoons in the freezer to apply to the eyes if they are swollen when getting up in the morning.

Before having any medical procedure done, know the cost, the possible side effects, and the downtime.

A doctor who guarantees results is an artist—con artist.

Read every medical permit before you sign, no matter how simple or how complicated. Questions? *Ask.*

Look at before and after photos of the procedure you are considering, and be sure that they were done by the doctor you are considering.

When having pictures taken for before and after procedures, find out what they are going to be used for and give your permission only if you agree.

Ointments have some occlusive effect on the skin and get moisture and active ingredients in better than creams.

Lotions are mostly creams with water added.

The reason you should not use adult topical products on children is not that they would penetrate deeper, but the smaller the child, the greater the relative surface area of skin, so they can get too great a dose.

Never share your prescription medicines (pills, capsules, creams, etc.) with anyone.

Make a copy of your passport, and put it in a safe place that you take with you in case you lose the original

Never give up your passport to anyone but a government official in a foreign country.

The leading cause of death in women in the US is the same as in men—heart disease.

Although a doctor may use a computer image to show you what can be done with a procedure, no doctor can match the results that a computer will show.

Coenzyme Q (CoQ10) plays a very important role in the function of the body but is too unstable to do anything in cosmetic preparations.

Looking for reviews of products from consumers? Go to www. makeupalley.com.

Products containing ground up apricot pits are actually very good exfoliators.

Facial mud masques are helpful in reducing oil and the size of pores. Ahava from the Dead Sea is an excellent one.

If lipstick runs up into the lines above your lips, Botox or Restylane can be used to help the problem.

If you pluck your eyebrows, do so before bedtime so that any redness will be gone by morning.

Restylane, Juvéderm, or similar hyaluronic acid products can be injected to form an internal lip liner to accentuate the lips without making them bigger.

Most caviar products for skin care are actually extracts and are heat processed, not pure, like the difference between eggs and scrambled eggs.

The food with the best source of antioxidants is broccoli sprouts.

Part of your daily routine should be a scheduled relaxation—yoga, stretching, or just sitting with your eyes closed while listening to music.

There are a number of forms of botulinum toxin available, and in the US, there are three that are effective and are proven safe: Botox˚, Dysport˚, and Xeomin˚.

Botulinum injections can be used and are approved for decreasing excess sweating under the arms or on the palms.

Perlane is a more robust and longer lasting form of Restylane which is available in the US, particularly good for scars or making lips bigger or fuller.

Despite all the marketing, no one can determine what type of skin you have and what you need without seeing you.

You may think your feet are getting bigger as you age. They are! From constant weight over the years, they do get wider.

Beware of before and after pictures as gospel; they are very easy to fake.

Products claiming to contain DNA probably don't, and if they do, provide no benefit for the skin at all.

Products from seaweed and algae do have great moisturizing benefits.

Gingko biloba has not been clinically shown to have benefit either when taken or applied.

"As seen on TV" means nothing except it was seen on TV.

A great inexpensive exfoliant is a paste made of cornmeal and water.

The best hand cream I have found is the one made by RoC.

To increase the strength and beauty of your nails, take grape-seed extract daily.

There are new skin-care products being developed from soy and other plants for their estrogen effects to reverse the effects of menopause on the skin.

For vaginal itching, do not douche with baking soda. Use a solution of one tablespoon white vinegar to a pint of water.

If taking antibiotics, eat cultured yogurt to avoid getting a yeast infection.

The only thing that will really help sagging skin of the face is a face-lift. All the rest is hype.

To avoid vitamin D deficiency, get sun in the early morning or late afternoon with no sunscreen applied.

Use alcohol to wipe the seat and arms of the airplane when you get on the plane, especially the tray.

Do take into account windchill factor or heat index when exercising or working outside.

If your doctor gives you a complete exam with your clothes still on, change doctors.

Take one day a week to eat or drink whatever you want.

When you first awaken, smile and thank God for the day. It will make every day better regardless of what happens.

Be suspicious of doctors' offices where the plants are dying.

Think about it—which do you take better care of: your car or your body?

Sign your organ donor card.

Have a living will and someone appointed to make health care decisions if you cannot make them.

Vitamin F is not really a vitamin but two essential fatty acids.

Essential fatty acids keep cell membranes healthy and also keep the immune system working properly.

Vitamin H or Biotin plays an important role in maintaining healthy hair.

Melasma or the mask of pregnancy occurs not only from pregnancy but also from birth control pills. Once established, it must be treated to improve. It will not go away at the end of pregnancy or stopping birth control pills.

Massive doses of vitamins not only are not beneficial, but some studies indicate they can be very dangerous.

For good mental and physical health, keep close to your family, hold on to your friends, and increase the circle of friends.

Periodontal health is not only important for dental hygiene but can prevent significant infections systemically. See your dentist every six months!

Increasing fiber in your diet not only keeps digestion on track but also decreases absorbed fat as fiber in the gut soaks up fat.

Do not take hormones from the health food store. There are no studies confirming their benefits, and they may be harmful.

On average, married men live about eleven months longer than single men. There is no increase in longevity for married women.

Volunteering to help others increases your self-worth.

You are never too old to become physically active. Benefits have been shown to occur in those taking up aerobic activity in their nineties.

Resistance training such as lifting weights is important to overall health just as aerobic exercise is.

Fillers can be used to correct the hollow look under the eyes, but be sure you choose someone very experienced in the procedure.

If you want to see how much gravity has affected your appearance, lie on the bed with your face off the side, and look into a mirror!

When performed properly, yoga releases endorphins just like running and getting a high.

It may be boring, but the best way to get washboard abs is Pilates.

Stress incontinence (leaking urine when sneezing or coughing) is not uncommon in women as they get older and have children. There is nonsurgical treatment available from a urologist.

Many plastic and cosmetic surgeons refuse to perform procedures on smokers due to the lack of oxygen getting to the skin.

There are many strange regulations on chemicals. Hydroquinone (a bleaching agent) is allowed up to 2 percent as a cosmetic in the US. 4 percent is a drug. It is banned in Japan.

Rhinoplasty (nose job) is the most difficult cosmetic procedure to perform. Seek out the doctor who corrects other doctor's mistakes.

Omega 3 and Omega 6 are essential fatty acids, i.e., they must be obtained from diet or supplements like vitamins and are important in cardiovascular health and the immune system.

Cold water fish like salmon and mackerel are the best source of omega fatty acids.

Most caviar skin-care products only contain heat-processed caviar extract. Mirra from Moscow contains cold-processed pure caviar. The difference—eggs versus scrambled eggs.

Weight gain or weight loss takes time to show up after changing an eating pattern, so give at least a week before deciding if something is not working.

No matter how strict you remain on a program, you will reach a point of leveling off in which nothing changes. This is temporary and normal. Continue with your program and do not be discouraged.

If a scar is white, the only treatment is to tattoo the area using the color of the surrounding skin.

Never stop taking any prescription medicine without your doctor's instruction. Do not even attempt to change the dosage. This could kill you.

If a tablet is scored, you can (if instructed to do so) cut it in half. If it is not or if it is a capsule, you cannot be certain as to exactly where the medication is. It may not be evenly distributed.

Take a week off and go to a destination spa for your vacation; it will provide value for the other fifty-one weeks of the year.

To try to take the spa experience home with you. Keep a diary while at the spa with your thoughts and feelings as you go through each day. Read it frequently when you get home.

Data showing studies reducing appearances of wrinkles, etc. may or may not be valid. Most experts can design studies to show almost anything. See what it does for *you*.

The number one product recommended by dermatologists for skin care is Cetaphil® because it causes no problem and is fragrance free.

Articles appearing in well-known and respected magazines dealing with health and beauty are generally well researched by the author and editors and have correct information.

Making a to-do list for the day? Put some time for yourself on it. Schedule for yourself.

Vegetarian sources for omega 3 include flaxseed, canola oil, walnuts, and leafy greens.

One food with a negative calorie deficit, i.e., requires more calories to eat than it contains—celery.

When buying a self tanner, look for DHA (dihydroxyacetone) and/or erythrulose as ingredients. These have been shown to be effective and safe.

The best method of applying self tanner is to use a scrub cleanser in the shower. Apply evenly to moist skin, pat dry, and wash your hands.

Use a tinted sunscreen with an A and B block on your face under your foundation. Foundation alone is not enough protection.

When you see a spokesperson on TV and you want to look like her, remember, she just spent over two hours in makeup.

Cellulite is not fat accumulation but is actually a blood vessel problem in response to female hormone.

Cellulite does not have to look like cottage cheese; it can be a rippling effect of the skin of the legs and buttocks.

Topical vitamin K has been shown to improve the redness associated with rosacea.

Most of the medicines used to treat rosacea are decades old and not particularly effective.

Cellulite affects no less than 80 percent and perhaps as much as 95 percent of women.

Human papilloma virus, which causes venereal warts, has been shown to contribute to the development of cervical cancer.

The country rated as healthiest in the world is Japan.

At the end of 2005, there were approximately forty million people in the world living with HIV.

Worldwide, only one in ten persons infected with HIV has been tested.

There is a blood test for the gene responsible for certain types of breast cancer to determine your susceptibility.

Pharmacists are not licensed to dispense prescription medications without a physician's prescription or authorization.

Want to live longer and enjoy it in the process? Want to see the face of God? Love someone!

THE SOCIETIES

If you think the battle in the media is hot, you should see what is going on behind the scenes! The desire to protect one's turf, which really translates into protecting income, is being fought on every level and is unbelievably rancorous. The American Academy of Cosmetic Surgery came into existence almost twenty years ago, comprised of physicians from many different specialties, all of whom had an interest in the cosmetic aspect of medicine. These doctors who were dermatologists, surgeons, ob-gyn, and many others came together in a forum of academics to learn and teach one another about what can be done to benefit the many patients seeking cosmetic procedures. This society met resistance from the American Society of Plastic Surgeons (at the beginning, known as the American Society of Plastic and reconstructive surgeons) to the point of ridicule and ostracism. Members of the AACS, even though they were knowledgeable, well-trained, and becoming more so every year, were met with derision and ridicule because they weren't real plastic surgeons and therefore could not have any expertise in the area of cosmetic surgery and cosmetic procedures.

Over the years, the AACS continued not only to have seminars and taught hundreds of physicians but also established both fellowships and board certification in cosmetic surgery. This is important in many aspects, not just to have another plaque on the wall but to prove expertise and proficiency in the knowledge and procedures that patients desire. Medical board specialty certification is a complicated area, but suffice it to say that there are nineteen criteria established by the American Board of Medical Specialties and the American Medical Association for a group to be certified. The AACS continued to educate, to persevere, and met all the criteria to become a recognized board; *but* the American Board of Medical Specialties would not recognize them. It actually took a lawsuit and a court order by the California courts to finally certify that all the criteria had been met and the American Board of Cosmetic Surgery could finally claim its rightful status. Is all of this in the best interest of the patient? I don't think so!

There is another battle being fought more recently, and again, this is meeting resistance on the battlefield of the turf, and that is the

American Academy of Aesthetic Medicine. This unique society can trace its origins back to Europe in the 1980s when a number of physicians came together to form an educational group of doctors interested in the aesthetic aspect of medicine. Under the leadership of Dr. Michel DeLune of Belgium and the United States, this led to a thriving society that instructs physicians all over the world on how to evaluate the aging face and body and how to treat it from all aspects. This society has only one requirement for attendance, and that is that the member be a licensed physician in any specialty. Internists, obstetricians, surgeons, emergency room doctors—everyone is coming together in a forum of learning and hands-on workshops to learn from the world's experts in each field how to best treat their patients. Is this in the patient's best interest? Of course it is. Is it in the best interests of plastic surgeons, dermatologists, or the societies that represent them? Perhaps not. But it is absolutely necessary to train doctors from multiple specialties to be able to treat their aesthetic patients, and we in the society learn from one another because everyone has a different perspective and brings something to the table.

This society is still in its infancy as far as the American Academy of Aesthetic Surgery is concerned, now entering its fifth year, but over the next several years, it will be certifying doctors in all aspects of aesthetic medicine and aesthetic surgery; and although the doctors will all be well trained and bring a multidisciplinary approach to the care of their patients, they will meet the same brick wall when the time comes to become a society with its own board of medical specialties.

INDEX

A

acid 6, 8, 26, 29, 32, 34, 36, 38, 39, 40, 42, 48, 49, 50, 51, 52, 53, 90, 92, 93, 96, 102, 105, 106
    alpha hydroxy 32, 36, 38, 53
    glycolic 32, 36, 37, 42, 52, 93, 96,
    hyaluronic 48, 49, 50, 51, 92, 96, 103
    lactic 36, 49, 50, 51, 96
    salicylic 38, 53
    tartaric 36, 52, 53
acne 38, 53, 55, 70, 94, 98, 99
aestheticians 13, 18, 33, 36, 52, 72, 74, 76, 79, 81, 87
aesthetic medicine 2, 66, 84
Aesthetic Medicine 78, 86, 110
Aesthetic Surgery 110
aging 1, 2, 5, 6, 7, 8, 9, 10, 12, 13, 14, 15, 17, 19, 22, 26, 32, 35, 42, 46, 54, 62, 73, 76, 81, 91, 94, 98, 99, 110
    appearance of 8, 12, 13, 29, 33, 37, 38, 47, 48, 50, 59, 61, 94, 97, 98, 99
    intrinsic 9, 94
    true 9, 12, 15, 16, 25, 26, 27, 33, 41, 46, 52, 55, 56, 57, 58, 59, 62, 63, 69, 73, 76, 80, 85, 93, 94, 96, 99
alcohol 8, 98
alkali 52, 102
allergies 87, 90
American Academy of Cosmetic Surgery 78, 109
American Academy of Plastic Surgeons 84
American Board of Medical Specialties 78, 85, 86, 109
American Board of Plastic Surgeons 14
Americans 4, 5, 40, 61, 63, 74, 82, 102
American Society of Plastic Surgeons 109
anesthesia 43, 55, 56, 86, 87
antioxidants 6, 89, 98, 104
Appearance International 82, 84
Artefill 50
aspirin 32, 53, 91, 101

B

baby boomers 1, 2, 26, 40, 73
birth control pills 105
blood thinners 32, 33
board certification 17, 56, 85, 109
Botox 10, 12, 15, 16, 17, 19, 20, 46, 47, 48, 66, 72, 75, 76, 78, 80, 92, 93, 94, 99, 104
bruising 32, 33, 47, 73, 94
Bruising 45
burning spectrum 61, 62

C

California 61, 80, 81, 109
CALIFORNIA 80
cancer 2, 7, 12, 15, 40, 61, 62, 91, 92, 94, 97, 98, 100, 108
Captique 50, 51
Cardinal Health 27, 33
cells 27, 28, 29, 36
cellulite 45
Cellulite 98, 107, 108
chemical peels 15, 18, 36, 52, 53, 54, 79, 80, 93, 102
Chemical peels 98
citric acid 36
clinics 83
collagen 12, 18, 19, 22, 28, 37, 48, 49, 50, 59, 60, 92, 97
Collagen 82, 95
complexion problems 7, 53, 94
concentrations 25, 28, 38, 53
cosmeceuticals 8, 30, 41, 64, 76, 89, 95, 112
cosmetic companies 13, 29, 100
cosmetic industry 18, 25, 34, 42, 64, 94, 95
cosmetic procedures 2, 3, 17, 66, 72, 73, 78, 79, 80, 82, 83, 85, 94, 109
cosmetic products 3, 95
cosmetics 8, 25, 37, 41, 42, 64, 66, 93, 96
cosmetic surgeons 14, 65, 86, 106
cosmetic surgery 2, 20, 21, 22, 66, 73, 79, 80, 82, 83, 86, 96, 109
Cosmetic Surgery 78
Costa Rica 82, 83
creams 8, 25, 26, 40, 100, 103

D

death 32, 56, 96, 103
Dermabrasion 15, 55

dermatologists 2, 7, 15, 22, 23, 25, 26, 33, 38, 40, 53, 62, 70, 72, 73, 78, 83, 107, 109, 110
dermatology 13, 15, 56, 78, 84, 85, 86
dermis 9, 27, 28
diet 5, 57, 98, 101, 105, 106
diseases 16, 40
doctors 2, 13, 14, 16, 17, 18, 19, 21, 22, 23, 24, 25, 34, 45, 46, 48, 57, 65, 66, 72, 73, 74, 76, 78, 80, 83, 84, 85, 93, 96, 100, 105, 109, 110
drugs 8, 19, 25, 27, 40, 41, 62, 64, 66, 70, 96
Duke University 29, 97, 98

F

face-lift 4, 7, 8, 11, 15
facials 17, 18, 72
fat 8, 9, 11, 26, 31, 45, 56, 57, 98, 101, 105, 106, 107
FDA 8, 19, 25, 26, 40, 41, 42, 46, 47, 48, 49, 50, 58, 61, 64, 65, 66, 80, 88, 95, 97, 98
fibers 12, 28, 49, 59, 95
fibroblast 28
filling materials 9, 11, 15, 17, 46, 48, 49, 50, 60, 64, 65, 66, 72, 73, 76, 80, 97
Florida 73
food 5, 36, 102, 104, 105, 107
foundation 96, 107
free radicals 6

G

gynecologists 2, 17, 21

H

hair 64, 93, 94, 100, 105
health care 20, 82, 105
heart bypass surgery 82, 83
HIV 62, 108
Hylaform 50

I

infomercials 13, 25, 68, 69, 94, 96
injections 12, 14, 15, 19, 22, 46, 47, 48, 49, 50, 65, 66, 78, 79, 92, 93, 94, 98, 99, 104

J

Johnson and Johnson 26, 41
Juvéderm Ultra 48, 50, 51

L

laser resurfacing 15
lipodissolve 45
liposuction 15, 56, 57
Liposuction 56, 96
liver 2, 8, 17, 20, 26, 27, 31, 32, 33, 34, 82, 92, 94

M

marketing 11, 13, 19, 22, 23, 25, 31, 34, 39, 45, 46, 59, 61, 67, 70, 74, 77, 89,
  93, 98, 100, 104
medical care 4, 19, 20, 82, 83, 84, 97
medical spas 38, 44, 72, 73, 74, 76, 79
medical tourism 82, 83
Medicare 16, 56, 87, 95
medicine 2, 13, 18, 19, 20, 53, 58, 61, 62, 66, 74, 79, 80, 84, 85, 86, 87, 97, 106,
  107, 109, 110
mesotherapy 45
microdermabrasion 55 95, 100
moisturizers 7, 36, 92, 96, 99
muscles 12, 46, 47, 92

N

Neutrogena Healthy Skin 28
nose 7, 10, 11, 12, 17, 47, 86, 106
nurse practitioners 18, 19, 20
nurses 18, 19, 22, 72, 73, 74, 76

O

oil gland 38, 53
ophthalmologists 15, 46
over-the-counter drugs 40, 41

P

para-aminobenzoic acid 40
Perlane 50, 51, 104
permanent 49
permanent filler 50, 65
pH 52, 53, 90, 102
plastic surgeons 2, 14, 15, 22, 23, 31, 33, 56, 72, 74, 78, 83, 110
Plastic surgeons 14, 23, 97
Plastic Surgeons 84, 109
pregnancy 93, 101, 105
prescription 25, 38, 64, 95, 100, 103, 106, 108

Q

Quintessence 30

R

Radiesse 49, 50, 98
Renova 26, 95
Restylane 20, 49, 51, 65, 92, 97, 103, 104
retinol 26, 27, 28, 37, 92, 93, 97, 98, 99, 102,
rosacea 98, 107

S

scars 28, 31, 50, 55, 92, 98, 99, 104
Sculptra 49, 50, 51, 93
self-esteem 3, 4, 6, 97, 99
skin cancer 7, 15, 22, 40, 61, 62, 91, 97, 100
skin care 13, 14, 25, 28, 68, 71, 73, 97, 100, 104, 107
skin care products 12, 14, 22, 83, 95, 96
skin cells 27
Skinceuticals 28
SkinMedica 28
skin tests 48
skin vitamin 28
sleep lines 9, 10, 93
SPF 41, 91, 92
stress 9, 50, 58, 98, 102
sunburn 40, 61, 91, 99
sunscreens 7, 40, 41, 90
surgery 2, 3, 14, 15, 16, 20, 21, 22
surgical procedures 22, 23, 72

T

tanning bed industry 61, 62, 63
tanning beds 61, 62, 63
Tanning beds 91
Tennessee 18
Thermage 59, 60
topical agents 32, 33, 59
topical vitamin 30, 32, 33, 47, 92, 93, 97, 102, 107

U

UVA 41, 61, 62, 63, 91
UVB 41, 61, 62, 63

V

W